Workouts for

Seniors

Over 60

Volume 1

*Guided Home Exercise Routines
to Improve Core Strength, Build
Balance, & Increase Energy*

By Iann M. Eckhardt

Contents

A FREE GIFT TO ALL MY READERS!

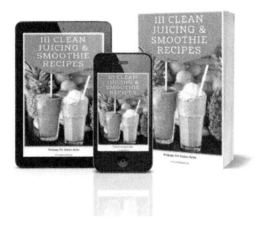

As a thank you, and to help you combine healthy nutrition with your exercise routines to maximize your results, I would like to send you a free copy of my fully illustrated eBook which contains 111 delicious juice and smoothie recipes that you can make at home!

To get your free copy now, please visit:

www.ianneckhardt.com

Introduction

Y ou walk into a room and forget why you came there. The stairs to the second level in your house have started to leave you breathless. You used to be able to open any jar with no problem at all. The pain in your joints has steadily worsened until you find your range of motion impaired and your independence threatened. I imagine that you picked up this book because you are seeing and feeling the signs of aging, and you want to do something about them. I am here to help!

My name is Iann Eckhardt, and I got into senior fitness when my mother developed pain and reduced mobility due to age, osteoporosis, and scoliosis. Using my ten years of experience in personal training, both one-on-one and in groups, I designed a fitness routine and nutrition regimen for my mom that helped lessen her pain, strengthen her muscles, and improve her overall well-being. But my mom is only one person. I have seen the effects of aging on a wide range of people, and it occurred to me that I could help a lot more people than just my mom and immediate clients, friends and family. That's why I wrote this book.

Helping you achieve the best possible results matters deeply to me. What you will learn in this book includes not only exercise routines targeted to seniors with your specific needs, but also information on the muscles in your body and what happens to them as you age. I believe that understanding the root of the problem is the first step to correcting it. Muscle loss due to aging, as you will find out in Chapter 1, is a natural process. It can't be stopped, but it can be slowed down. Being at your physical best will help you live a longer, healthier, and more rewarding life. Because of my mom and my experience helping her, this topic has become my passion.

How to use this book.

Begin by reading Chapter 1 to learn what happens to your body during the aging process starting when you are in your mid-30s. This general introduction to muscle groups, deterioration caused by aging, and methods for stopping or reversing the damage through core training and nutrition, is essential for understanding the mission you are on to improve your health and lessen your pain.

Chapter 2 contains your warmup routine plus guidelines for getting maximum benefit from the workout chapters. Since you should always warm up before working out, it is important not to skip this chapter. After these first two chapters, you can read the rest of the book straight through or go directly to workouts targeted at areas of your greatest interest or need. All workout routines have clear, step-by-step instructions and illustrations. In the end, you will be able to build your own workout plan by combining routines that target different muscle groups in the body. Guidelines for doing this are provided in the conclusion.

Therefore, for example, if your major complaint is joint pain and stiffness, you can start with Chapter 8, but if you really want to get to work on those arms, you can go directly to Chapter 4. I recommend designing an exercise plan that works all muscle groups at least once a week.

Some general guidelines for working out.

1. Wear breathable clothing and sturdy athletic shoes with support.

2. Keep water nearby and stop for a sip often. I recommend ice-cold water because studies have shown that it keeps you 50% more hydrated than cool or warm water and allows you to exercise longer (Barnett, n.d.).

3. If you eat before working out, wait at least a half hour! The old rule is true. Exercising on a full stomach can cause reflux, make you feel nauseous, or even give you the hiccups! Besides that, after you eat, your body increases blood flow to your digestive system. When you exercise, you want all of that blood going to your muscles.

4. Do less and gain more! Follow the instructions for each exercise and remember that you get twice the benefit from doing the exercise correctly. You can

actually exercise less and see better and faster results if you take the time to do it right.

5. Pay attention to form and breathing. Don't discount the very real benefits of following the guidelines for breathing in each exercise. You employ a very large muscle (the diaphragm) every time you take a breath. Since you have to breathe while you exercise, you might as well mindfully engage that muscle and reap the rewards—again, doing less and gaining more.

6. Listen to your body. While there are some exceptions, most of the exercises can be done seated or standing. Depending on your personal fitness level, choose which is better for you. Never push yourself into pain. You are working out to alleviate pain!

Finally, I'd like to remind you that you get a free, full-color, illustrated booklet filled with recipes for healthy juices and smoothies along with the purchase of this book. It's my way of saying thank you and encouraging you to combine good nutrition with your exercise adventure.

Ready to feel better, stronger, faster? Let's get started!

CHAPTER 1

Core Strength and the Aging Process

O ur muscles. They range from the tiniest one in the ear (stapedius), to the largest one on the rear (gluteus maximus), to the strongest one in the jaw (masseter). Kind of sounds like "mass eater," doesn't it? Anatomists classify these muscles in too many ways to explain here, so we will stick to the basic information we need to understand what our muscles do and why.

Muscles protect. Strong muscles protect and buttress our bones, joints, and internal organs. They absorb shocks to the body, like falls and bumps, to protect us from breaks and internal injuries. When these muscles are weak, it can lead to problems such as breaks, friction in the joints, or organ problems, such as weak bladder.

Muscles stabilize. Strong muscles allow us to balance and maintain good posture. For good posture, we need muscles that are both strong and flexible. Good posture is important because when we get into the habit of poor posture, it leads to pain. This pain can pop up anywhere, but it is most common in the back, neck, and shoulders.

Muscles regulate. Of course, we know that the heart is the most important muscle for circulation, but did you know that our muscles help regulate respiration, digestion, and excretion? Muscles also monitor body temperature. The majority of heat generated by the body comes from the contraction of muscles. That is why, when we are cold, it helps to get up, move around, and generate some heat. If we don't, the muscles will try and do it without our help—by shivering!

Muscles move. From the smallest movement of the eye to the most energetic movement of our running legs, strong and flexible muscles allow us freedom to move when and where we will. When our muscles are not strong, our freedom of movement is limited. That is not a pleasant feeling, I'm sure you will agree. Our muscles take care of the first three items on this list without our conscious thought. However, when our muscles are not there for us when we want to move, or lift, or bend, or reach—we know about it right away. And we don't like it.

At birth, our muscles are programmed to grow larger and stronger. That is why kids can eat peanut butter and jelly and drink soda pop and still be strong, flexible, and active (oh, so active!) Around early middle-age, however, that program starts to shut down. This usually starts happening sometime in a person's thirties. Adults begin to lose muscle mass, and, instead of being used for building more muscle, peanut butter and jelly is converted into fat. Unfortunately, no matter what we do, we begin to lose muscle and gain fat. Even if we are active, this natural, biological process is going to occur. It is called sarcopenia.

Sarcopenia simply means natural loss of muscle tissue due to the aging process. It is not some terrible disease, but the more sedentary we are, the greater the loss of muscle mass and so the greater our difficulty (or pain) in doing the things we enjoy. The process begins in our thirties, fat invades our muscles starting in our fifties, and the process increases more rapidly in our sixties and beyond.

Causes of sarcopenia include age, changes in hormone levels, changes in protein conversion, changes in our cells, and inflammation. Factors that contribute to how quickly and how profoundly sarcopenia affects us include inactivity or lack of exercise, prolonged bed rest, loss of mobility, poor nutrition, and obesity. Chronic diseases, such as diabetes, arthritis, heart disease, and gastrointestinal disorders, can also speed up this natural process (*Sarcopenia*, n.d.).

We are here because we want to slow it down.

Some of the effects of sarcopenia:

- Difficulty with daily activities

- Impaired balance and the ability to walk, leading to falls and fractures

- Muscles no longer protect bones and joints as effectively, leading to injury

- Increased fatigue

- Higher risk of disease

- Existing, chronic conditions can worsen

- Weight gain

- Loss of mobility and/or independence

- Diminished quality of life

We can ask our physician to help us gauge how advanced our sarcopenia is. Generally, they will subject us to what is called the SARC-F Test. Our sarcopenia can be diagnosed as advanced based on these markers.

S — stands for strength. Patient cannot lift and carry ten pounds.

A — stands for assistance. Patient needs help walking across a room.

R — stands for rising. Patient has difficulty getting up from a chair or a bed

C — stands for climbing. Patient has difficulty climbing ten or more stairs.

F — stands for falls. Patient has fallen within the past year.

Depending on answers and abilities, doctors can determine how advanced a patient's sarcopenia is. No matter how weak we may feel we have become, there is something we can do about it. And even if we are only starting to feel those effects now, we can slow down the process!

Three types of muscle. Let's talk about our muscles some more. We have three types of muscle in our bodies.

Cardiac muscles, or heart muscles, are involuntary, which means that they work on their own without our conscious help.

Smooth muscles are also involuntary. They are found in the walls of our hollow organs (like the stomach).

Skeletal muscles are attached to our bones by tendons. They are under voluntary control, which means that we can decide to move them, or not. We can decide to strengthen them, or not. We can work with them to make them more flexible, or not. Happily, if you are reading this book, that "or not," does not apply to you!

Core muscles are the muscles that connect to and support our spine and our hips. Prioritize strengthening our core muscles, and all of our other muscles benefit, too. As an added bonus, studies have shown that resistance training is also effective in fighting cognitive decline, which usually starts as confusion and memory loss as early as age 45 (Nagamatsu, 2012). The workout chapters of this book will address each of these core muscle groups:

- Transverse abdominis—part of the "abs" that directly affects the lower back and hips

- Internal and external obliques—the inner and outer layers of abdominal muscles on our sides

- Rectus abdominis—the part of the abdominals that we usually think of when we say "abs"

- Erector spinae—the deep muscles of the back that extend from the skull to the pelvis

- Diaphragm—large muscle beneath the lungs that expands and contracts as we breathe

- Pelvic floor muscles—provide support for the pelvic organs (bowel and bladder)

- Minor core muscles—trapezius (traps/upper back), latissimus dorsi (lats/middle back), and gluteus maximus (hips/lower back).

All of the muscles of the body work together — everything is connected. Think of your core as the central command. A strong and flexible central command will support any and all movement in the extremities. This is why it is important to work your core during every exercise session. There is more than one way to do this, so if you're saying to yourself, "Oh, great, here come the crunches," you can relax. In fact, go ahead and laugh. Strong, deep belly laughter is a *great* workout for your core muscles!

Core Muscles, Health, and You

Imagine a ballerina dancing on stage. Ballet dancers have some of the strongest cores on Earth. The torso is lifted, and every movement originates in the dancer's core. The arms and legs are extensions of the core. Core strength, even more than artistic skill, is what gives a dancer power and grace.

The exercises in the coming chapters will address core strength and flexibility. In turn, core strength will improve your balance, mobility, energy, and overall feeling of wellbeing. You should also experience a lessening of pain and greater freedom of movement.

It does not matter how old you are. The younger you are when you start exercise targeted toward delaying the effects of aging, the more you can stave them off. If you are in your forties and starting to see the effects of sarcopenia (increased belly fat, for example, that has started accumulating even though you haven't changed your eating or exercise habits since you were twenty), you can start today and get out in front. If you are in your fifties and experiencing annoying memory problems that you never had before along with increased weight and decreased strength, you can start today and begin to reverse the effects of sarcopenia. If you are in the over 60 crowd, you can start today to *reverse the effects* of aging, decrease your aches and pains, and improve your mobility *even if you can check all of the boxes on the SARC-F Test.*

The most important thing is that now you know what is causing the problem. And this book is your key to changing yourself for the better.

Let's try a little experiment. Reach out in front of you, like you're going to grab something floating in the air. Close your fist around that invisible object and then pull your arm back. Do that a couple of times. Great! Hopefully, that was a simple movement and easy for you to complete.

Now, do it again, but this time notice which muscles you engage as you reach out and bring your arm back to your side. Did you do it? If so, you probably felt your arm muscles as you extended your hand, the muscles in your hand as you closed your fist, and maybe even the muscles in your back directly behind your outstretched arm. Because it is such a simple movement, you might not have felt the involvement of your abdominals, but it was there.

When you think of working from your core, imagine that it is centered at your belly button. You are going to reach out and perform the same movement that you did before, but *this time* you will actively engage your core. This will require you to *think first* and then move. Imagine that the command to reach out and grab that invisible treat is coming from your core, your command center, instead of your brain. Your belly button is pushing your hand out into space. You will have to think first in order to pass the command from your brain, to your core command center, and then out to your arm and hand. Give it a try. What did you feel?

If the movement originated in your core, you should have felt your belly button move back toward your spine as you reached out and grasped and then relax as you pulled your arm back to your side. Did you feel it? Try it again. You just worked your core in a very simple way by moving your hand.

When you do the upcoming exercises, be mindful of transferring command from your brain to your core. Any movement that originates from the core will be 1) more complete, 2) easier to perform, 3) twice as beneficial.

Why is that? Well, reach out with just your hand again; then, reach out with your hand *from your core command center.* Do you feel the difference? When you only reach out with your hand, you engage smaller muscle groups. However, when you reach out from your core, you fully engage large muscle groups. You might even have noticed a slightly elevated heart rate from the core-commanded motion.

The lesson here is that you can work your core no matter what you do. Washing dishes? Put your core in charge. Mowing the lawn? Push that mower with your belly button. And absolutely fully engage your core as you do every exercise and workout in this book. You will see twice the results in half the time. Engaging the core command center is a mind-body connection that you consciously make, and you can do it when you are fully relaxed, too. Just imagine that your core is watching that television show or enjoying that hot bath. The more you do this, the more you strengthen that connection, and then moving from your core will gradually become a good habit. Habits are things we do without thinking about them. To create that habit, however, we have to pay attention and do it mindfully at first.

The upcoming exercises will fall into three categories:

1. Stretching the muscles for flexibility

2. Contracting the muscles for strength

3. Cardio to boost the immune system and improve circulation

Feed your muscles: A word about nutrition

While this book is primarily an exercise guide, we need to remember that any exercise regime goes hand-in-hand with proper nutrition. Recall that one of the causes of sarcopenia is the body's changing ability to process the proteins we eat into the proteins our bodies use to function. For seniors with inflammation, the foods you eat can have a significant impact on the amount of joint and back pain you feel.

Because of this, I'm going to give you some lists of the five best and worst foods to eat to combat inflammation. They are, also, the best and worst in general. Whether or not you currently have the aches and pains associated with inflammation, the general degeneration of the spine begins at the same time as sarcopenia. This makes sense because the muscles that support the spine become weaker, leaving the bones less protected. According to the World Health Organization, 60%-70% of people experience lower back pain, and it only gets worse as we age. The old-timers used to call it *lumbago*. No matter what we call it, we new-timers will experience it, too. The items on the list come from the researchers at Harvard Medical School (Harvard Health Publishing, 2018).

The Five Worst Foods for Inflammation

1. Refined carbohydrates—breads, cakes, cookies, potato chips, etc.

2. Fried foods

3. Sugar—any food or beverage with sugar or high fructose corn syrup

4. Meat—red meats and processed meats (hot dogs, cold cuts, sausage)

5. Fat—margarine, shortening, and lard

The Five BEST Foods to Fight Inflammation

1. Berries—all kinds plus cherries and oranges!

2. Green leafy veggies—especially broccoli, spinach, and Brussels sprouts

3. Fatty fish—tuna, salmon, mackerel, and sardines

4. Nuts—especially almonds and walnuts

5. Fat—olive oil

In addition, Harvard researchers recommend that seniors involved in strength training (that's you!) increase daily intake of natural proteins. Foods like lean chicken, salmon, Greek yogurt, skim milk, eggs, and cooked beans all made their list. As you can see, the foods that are good for you are readily available and generally not any more expensive than the foods that are harmful.

Before you begin using the exercises in this book, I recommend talking to your doctor about your plans. There is also no harm in talking to a nutritionist or dietician about the nutrients you need to replace as you increase your amount of normal activity.

Remember — you want to feed your muscles, and they do not crave junk food.

How exercise reduces body aches and pains

First, exercise releases endorphins, which are the human body's version of an opioid. Any type of exercise will release them (sex, dancing, drumming). We feel happier after these activities not only because we enjoy them but because after doing them, we are overrun by endorphins. Second, exercise builds the muscles that protect joint and nerve centers so that they can bed down, get comfortable, and stop crying. If we are sedentary, we do not get relief from pain in either of these ways. When it comes to the aches and pains of aging, studies cited by Harvard Medical School have shown that bedrest actually makes matters worse *(Bed rest for back pain? A little bit will do you., 2015)*. Becoming *more* active is the prescription for mitigating pain.

In addition, regular exercise has other health benefits for seniors that include helping to control blood pressure, reducing feelings of depression and anxiety, improving quality of sleep, and boosting feelings of wellbeing (HUR USA, n.d.).

In the *Physical Activity Guidelines for Americans 2nd Edition,* the U.S. Department of Health and Human Services recommends 2.5 to 5 hours of cardio per week plus two sessions per week of resistance training for all adults. For seniors, they recommend adding balance training as well (2018). Luckily for us, core training IS balance training.

Now, let's get to the workout!

CHAPTER 2

The Workout—Stretching

S tretching involves elongating muscle. When you think of stretching, imagine a rubber band. The rubber band will stretch just fine, but it wants to return to its resting length. Your muscles will want to do that, too. Stretch a rubber band too far, and it will break. There is no danger of that as long as you listen to your body and ease your stretch at the first sign of any pain. Feeling a slight *ache* in your muscles when you stretch is what you want to aim for.

Stretching can be a workout by itself because it improves flexibility and the range of motion in the joints. However, stretching should *always* precede any type of physical exercise because it prepares the body for the work ahead and decreases the risk of injury. Because more harm than good can result from stretching incorrectly, doctors at the Mayo Clinic recommend the following guidelines (Mayo Clinic Staff, 2017a).

Don't stretch cold. Warm up your muscles with a short walk, a dance around the living room, or a good laugh. The stretch routine provided below is intended to be a warmup for the core exercises that follow. Therefore, you can perform the stretch routine without a prior warm up.

Focus on symmetry. Most people have tighter muscles on one side of the body. You will probably find that you can stretch farther more easily on one side. That's great! It also means that you need to spend a little more time and effort on the other side. Being equally as strong and flexible on both sides helps with stability and balance.

Don't bounce! When you hold a stretch, never bounce. It does not make you more flexible, and bouncing can actually make muscles tighter rather than loosen and elongate them. Bouncing is bad.

Hold instead. Once you have reached that point in a stretch where you feel the slight ache that tells you your muscle is working, stop there and hold the stretch. The longer you hold the stretch, the greater the benefit. Instructions for what to do while holding a stretch will be given in the individual exercises.

Stretch regularly. The benefits of stretching will be lost if you don't stretch two or three times a week. Stretching can help you increase your range of motion, but those stubborn muscles will undo all that work if you stop. Unfortunately, they would rather be short rubber bands.

Mindful execution of stretch routines will help improve your flexibility, circulation, and posture. However, posture is another good habit you have to get into. Practicing good posture while you stretch is a great way to do this. Not paying attention to posture while you exercise will not improve your posture at all. So, let's talk about posture.

Posture

Imagine that you are nothing but a skeleton—all bones. Have a look at your spine. It runs the length of your core from your pelvis up into your skull. It is not straight—it has a natural curve. Your skull sits on top of it like the head on a bobble-head doll. Ready for another little experiment? Nod your skull back, tilting your chin toward the sky and then bring it back to center. Nod your skull down, tilting your chin toward your chest and then bring it back to center. Your skull is meant to sit comfortably on the top of your spine in a level way. *You cannot have good posture if your skull is out of place.*

Tilt your head back again and notice the *tension* at the base of your skull. Feel it? Good. Tilt your head forward again and notice the *stretch* in the muscles of your neck. It feels good to stretch those muscles, doesn't it? Adjust your head at the top of your spine so that you feel *no tension and no stretch*. This is proper alignment of the head. You will most likely feel that your chin is closer to your chest than usual. Most people live habitually with a slightly backward head tilt, which causes tension that leads to back and neck pain. Getting into the habit of proper alignment will alleviate that chronic pain! Want to check and see if you've got your skull on right? Grab the tops of your ears and pull straight up—your head should move into alignment as the tops of your ears point directly at the ceiling. Try that with your head tilted back. What happened? Your chin fell forward, didn't it?

Continue by imagining that you are a skeleton in a science classroom, and you are hanging from one of those science-classroom hooks. Your skull is at the proper angle, and your spine dangles. Now, mentally add your shoulder bones to your spine. Add your ribcage, surrounding your spine. Add your pelvic bones at the base of your spine. Hang your arm bones from your shoulders. Hang your leg bones from your pelvis. Have a look at perfect alignment. The arms and legs can swing freely. Everything is loose and full of space.

We have to attach muscle to those bones, but we want those bones to stay in perfect alignment when we set our feet on the floor or our bottom on a chair. Because of gravity, we can't just hang around in perfect alignment— our muscles have to hold us up. However, when you think of getting into alignment, *think of your bones first.*

So, what does "shoulders back and down" mean? When a person's habitual head tilt causes tension followed by pain, people try to mitigate that pain by *raising their shoulders* instead of adjusting the position of the head (which is the real problem). People generally also have a habit of *rolling their shoulders forward.* You want to get into the habit of rolling your shoulders back and letting them hang (as though you were all skeleton). You can roll them back easily enough (it's even part of the workout), but you cannot force them down. You have to *think them down.*

Sit or stand with your skull and spine in alignment—no tension, no stretch, tops of the ears pointed at the ceiling. Your arms should hang freely at your sides. If they cannot hang freely where you are sitting, then stand up for this. Gently roll your shoulders back a couple of times, coming to rest when you are sure they are not rolled forward. Close your eyes (after you finish reading this) and see the bottom of your earlobe and the top of your shoulder. Mentally, ask your earlobe and shoulder to move away from each other. In your imagination, watch your earlobe move up and your shoulder move down. Don't DO anything physically, but ALLOW for movement. You may feel nothing, or you may feel your shoulder relax a little, and you might even feel your shoulder drop a little. Give it a try on both sides.

Now, with your shoulders "back and down" gently move your head around. *Always be gentle with your neck and head.* You should feel a tad more freedom of movement than you are used to. If you hear a bit of popping and crackling, that is tension being released and fluid being redistributed.

Daily, mindful practice improving your posture can foster immediate and considerable results in easing chronic pain in your neck, shoulders, and back. Proper alignment is a must not just when exercising but every second of your day. It really is the one thing that can ease chronic neck and back pain immediately.

Most of the exercises in this book will direct you to "sit or stand in alignment." To stand in alignment, make sure your skull is sitting correctly and the rest of your bones are in the "hanging" position described above. Your toes should be pointing straight in front of you, neither angled inward nor outward. To sit in alignment, you should sit forward, more or less on the "edge of your seat," with your feet flat on the floor. From this position, you can check the alignment of your head and allow your arms to hang freely at your sides. You should use a sturdy chair that does not have armrests.

Warm up Stretch Routine

1. **Warm up your core using your diaphragm and abs**

The diaphragm is the large muscle beneath your lungs. You move it with your breath. This exercise will engage both your diaphragm and your abs. Deep Belly Breathing is a gentle and effective way to energize your core.

➢ Sit or stand in alignment.

➢ Imagine that your belly is a balloon.

➢ Breathe in deeply through your nose and direct all of that air into your belly balloon.

➤ Keep breathing in until there is absolutely no more room for any more air.

➤ Hold that breath for a count of two. Don't raise your shoulders!

➤ Release the air by blowing out your mouth.

➤ As you blow, press your belly button back toward your spine until there is absolutely no more air left to blow. Push, push, push that air out!

➤ Hold with no breath for a count of two.

➤ Release and treat yourself to two or three normal breaths; notice your heart rate and any other changes in how you feel.

➤ Repeat and hold for a count of four. Rest.

➤ Repeat and hold for a count of six. Rest.

➤ Repeat and hold for a count of eight. Rest.

If you can't hold your breath for a full eight counts at first, that's okay. Do what you can. You can work up to it! Don't forget to check your alignment before every inhale.

How do you feel? Ideally, you feel warmer all over, more relaxed, and ready for more.

2. Giant Arcs to Heaven

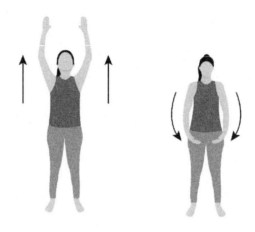

Let's add a feeling of flow to the breath. You will continue working your diaphragm, but you will not need to push with the abs. You do want to perform the exercise on the breath, however, because that is the element that engages the core.

➢ Sit or stand in alignment.

➢ As you breathe in, lift your straight arms out to your sides, palms up, all the way up until your palms meet over your head with your arms fully extended.

The amount of time that it takes your palms to meet overhead should be the same amount of time it takes you to breathe in fully through your nose.

Extend your arms energetically as you raise them and imagine that you are lifting something with a bit of weight (but not too much).

Your palms should meet as you finish your inhale.

> ➤ Turn your palms outward and lower your arms in the same arc as you blow out through your mouth.

Use your entire exhale to lower your arms.

Extend your arms energetically as you lower them and imagine that you are pushing something with a bit of resistance down.

> ➤ Allow your arms to fully relax as they reach the bottom; they will want to flop and cross each other a little as you prepare to breathe in and continue; let them!

> ➤ Repeat for a total of 8.

If eight repetitions is too much for you, start with four. When you are ready, go to six. Finally, build up to eight.

3. Neck Stretches

Always be gentle with your neck. Move slowly, and make sure you are in alignment before you move your head. Neck stretches will be most beneficial if you make sure you are in bobble-head position, so pull up on those ears first! While you are stretching, you might start to think that if you adjust your head position a little, you can stretch farther—*don't do it!* The better aligned you are, the more beneficial the stretch will be. Stretching "farther" while out of alignment is counterproductive.

4. Lean to the Side

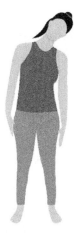 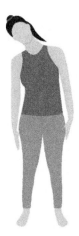

➢ Sit or stand in alignment.

➢ Gently lower your right ear toward your right shoulder.

➢ You will feel the stretch in the left side of your neck.

➢ Hold the stretch there as you take four, full relaxed breaths in and out through your nose.

➢ As you breathe, ask your left earlobe to move away from your left shoulder.

- ➢ Gently lift your head to center and take a couple of recovery breaths.

- ➢ Check your alignment and repeat on the other side.

- ➢ Repeat each side once more for a total of two times on each side.

Double check your alignment each time before you lower your head.

It's a good idea to close your eyes to imagine your earlobe and shoulder moving away from each other. Again, don't do anything to make this happen, just ask and imagine.

Try not to move anything but your head. Leaning to the side with your body will not increase the stretch in your neck.

5. Look to the Side

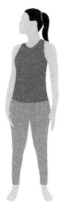 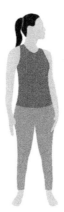

➢ Are you in alignment?

➢ Imagine that your nose is a piece of chalk preparing to draw an arc in the air.

➢ Keeping your chin level, gently follow your nose to the right until the stretch stops you.

➢ Hold the stretch there for two full relaxed breaths. On the exhales, encourage your nose to draw just the tiniest bit more of the arc toward your shoulder.

➢ Gently follow your nose back to center.

➢ Check your alignment and repeat on the other side.

➢ Repeat on each side once more for a total of two times on each side.

➢ Be mindful not to turn your body; just turn your head.

Deepening the stretch is what you do when you increase the stretch during an exhale. When you exhale, tell yourself to relax. If you relax when you exhale, you will find that your body will automatically increase the stretch a tiny amount. A tiny amount is the perfect amount. Always remember that you will get greater results from stretching if you mindfully relax. As you continue with the exercises, understand that deepen the stretch means inhale; as you exhale, consciously relax into the stretch; allow your body to respond by stretching a tiny bit farther on its own with each exhale.

6. Look Up and Down

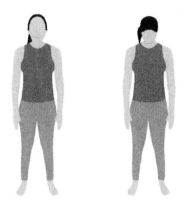

➤ Check your alignment.

➤ Slowly and gently, tilt your head back to look up.

➤ Stop when you feel the tension at the base of your skull and the stretch at your throat; you will not hang out here.

➤ Bring your head back to center.

➤ Gently lower your chin toward your chest.

➤ Allow your head to hang there for two full, deep breaths and deepen the stretch.

➤ Bring your head back to center and take a couple of recovery breaths.

➤ Repeat once.

7. Shoulder Blade Squeeze

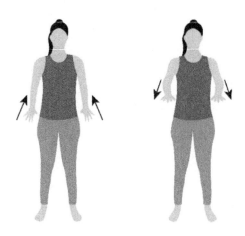

While this is not, strictly speaking, a stretch, it is good for warming up the shoulders and releasing tension in the back. It also helps with the "shoulders back and down" habit.

- ➤ Stand in alignment.
- ➤ Lift your shoulders up toward your ears as you inhale. UP.
- ➤ Move your arms back and press your shoulder blades together as you exhale. BACK.
- ➤ Allow your shoulders to relax down as you finish exhaling. DOWN.
- ➤ Repeat for a total of 8.

8. Alternating Giant Arm Circles

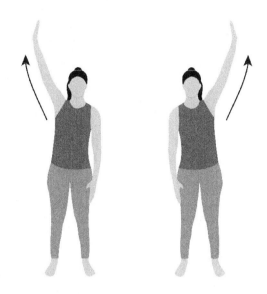

Let's do some big movement to open up the chest and lubricate the shoulders.

> ➢ Sit or stand in alignment with your arms hanging loosely at your sides.

> ➢ Engage your core by taking in a nice, deep breath through your nose.

> ➢ As you exhale, raise your right arm straight out in front of you like you were going to roll on a nice new wall paint.

> ➢ When your arm reaches the top, swing back and around, completing the circle.

> ➢ Complete the entire arm circle in the time it takes you to breathe out.

- ➤ Do the other arm on the next exhale.

- ➤ Alternate arms for a count of eight (four on each side).

You will probably find that one arm moves farther and more easily than the other. If that is the case, increase the number of circles on the weaker side to two. For example, Juliet is weaker on her left side, so she alternates 1 giant arm circle on the right with 2 giant circles on the left for a total of 12 (4 on the right and 8 on the left).

9. Washing Machine Gentle Cycle

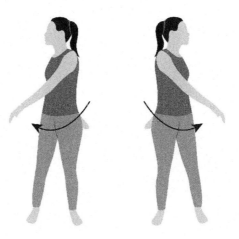

This warmup is the best of both worlds: it is very relaxing, and it gently warms up the abs and spine. Do it slowly.

➢ Stand in alignment with your arms hanging freely at your sides.

➢ Gently rotate your torso right and left, allowing your head to go with the motion.

➢ Count to twenty as you move (1=right, 2=left, 3=right, and so on).

As you rotate, you will notice that your arms start to follow the motion like swings on a turning carnival ride. Let them swing freely. They will probably start gently smacking into your belly and back as you reverse your rotation. Good! They are supposed to do that. Your arms should follow the movement of your torso like noodles.

Turn gently but fully. If you have lower back issues, you might hear a pop from that area. As long as there is NO PAIN along with the pop, the pop is good. It means you are releasing tension and redistributing fluid. Do not try to make your back pop. Just rotate gently and be mindful of staying in alignment.

10.Arm Swings with Fingers Laced

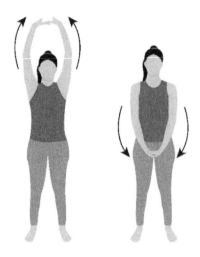

This warmup can be a little more challenging depending on your arm flexibility and strength. A modification will follow.

➤ Sit or stand in alignment.

➤ As you inhale, lift both arms straight out in front of you like you're holding and raising a baby.

➤ When your arms reach chest level, lace your fingers together with your fingers gripping the backs of your hands.

➤ As you exhale, bring your laced hands in toward your chest and then turn your palms over and press your laced hands down toward the floor (as in the illustration).

➤ As you inhale, arc your arms up over your head and turn your palms over to face the ceiling.

➤ Press your laced hands energetically toward the ceiling as you exhale.

➤ Inhale.

➤ As you exhale, release your fingers and lower your arms in the same manner as Giant Arcs to Heaven.

➤ Repeat for a total of four.

Modification—if you have difficulty keeping your fingers laced when you raise your hands over your head with your palms facing upward:

➤ Begin the same way - as if you are lifting a baby.

➤ When your arms reach chest level, lace your fingers the opposite way—so that your fingers are on the inside of your hands and touching the palms.

➤ Complete as above.

Lacing your fingers in the opposite way will make the exercise easier, and you can work up to doing it the regular way as you become stronger and more flexible.

11. Easy Side Stretch

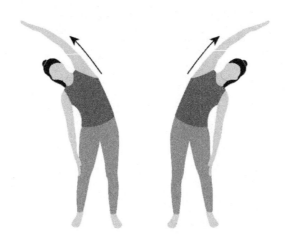

Alignment is key here. Yes, you will be able to stretch farther if you are not in alignment, but just think about that for a moment. If you can stretch farther while out of alignment, what you are doing is making it easier to feel good about *how far* you can stretch rather than getting the most effective stretch. Be very mindful of this, please.

➢ Sit or stand in alignment. If you are standing, give yourself a nice, wide stance to help with balance.

➢ Raise your right arm up over your head with your flat palm facing left. The inside of your right arm should be very close to your right ear, almost touching. At the same time, rest your left palm against the outside of your left leg.

➢ Inhale a nice, big, deep, breath.

➢ As you exhale: reach up toward the ceiling with your right hand and reach toward the floor with your left hand.

➢ Slide your left hand down the outside of your leg and allow your right arm to follow as you bend to the left, following your left hand.

➢ Stop when you feel a nice stretch in your right side.

➢ Deepen the stretch. Take two, full deep breaths while you hold the stretch. Remind yourself to relax so that you can allow your left hand to move just a tiny bit farther down your leg on both exhales.

➢ Inhale your third breath.

➢ As you exhale, reach energetically for the ceiling with your right hand and bring it in a rainbow arc back down to your side.

➢ Allow your torso to follow the movement of your right arm and come back to upright standing. Allow your left hand to slide back up your left leg.

➢ Repeat on the other side.

➢ Repeat both sides for a total of two stretches on each side.

Important—reach up with your raised hand BEFORE you start to bend.

Keep your attention on the hand that is sliding down the leg rather than on your raised arm.

Keep a stable base. DO NOT lock your knees. DO NOT pop your hip out to one side. Notice that in the illustration, the legs and hips remain straight and stable. Popping your hip out will give you the illusion that you are stretching farther, but it is VERY bad for your lower back.

The bigger belly breath you take, the better. When you breathe in while in this position, you will notice that the air is directed toward the stretched side. It cannot get into the other side because it is contracted. Therefore, just breathing while in the stretch increases the benefit even if your opposite hand does not move any farther down your leg.

It does not matter how far you stretch. What matters is feeling that ache in your side. For beginners, just reaching toward the ceiling is enough of a stretch at first. Listen to your body. Never force anything when stretching.

Relax and breathe

12. Opposite Presses

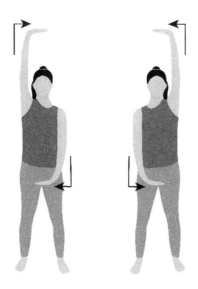

Let's follow that up with something that requires a little less effort. Breathing is key in this exercise!

➢ Sit or stand in alignment.

➢ As you inhale, raise your arms in front of you.

➢ Flex your hands.

➢ As you exhale, energetically press the palm of one hand toward the floor and the other toward the ceiling.

➢ Continue to press lightly as you inhale.

➢ Energetically press up and down as you exhale.

➢ Repeat for two more breaths (press for a total of three exhales).

- Lower your arms as you inhale.

- Repeat by reversing the palms (so that what went up goes down).

- After your last exhale, bring your hands back down to your sides.

You should feel this mostly in your upper arms, but you are also working on the flexion of your wrists and the strength in your hands.

13.Supported Hip Circles

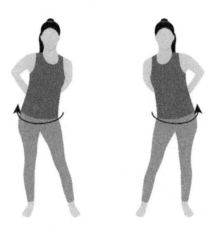

The size of the hip circles is not important. This exercise should feel good at your lower back. If you feel any pain or strain in your lower back, make your circle size smaller.

- Stand in alignment with your feet in a wide stance.

➢ Place your palms on your lower back, the heels of your hands at the bottom of your ribcage and the fingers pointing down on your hips.

➢ Gently circle your hips in one direction for a count of 8 circles.

➢ Gently circle in the other direction for another count of 8.

14. Hamstring Stretch

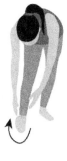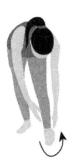

This exercise requires good balance. If you are worried about balance, do the exercise seated on a chair.

➢ Stand or sit in alignment.

➢ Take a big step forward with your right foot. (Extend your right leg out in front of you, if sitting).

➤ Your right foot needs to be flexed, so lift your toes and balance on your right heel.

➤ Keeping your left hand on your left thigh, bend your left knee.

➤ When you bend your knee, you will hinge forward at the hips.

➤ Reach for the toes of your right foot with your right hand as you exhale.

➤ Maintain that position as you inhale.

➤ Remind yourself to relax as you exhale. Try to get a tiny bit closer to your toes with your extended hand for a total of 4 exhales.

➤ Return to standing.

➤ Repeat on the other side.

It does not matter if you can't touch your toes. You want to feel that slight tightness in the back of your extended leg. Once you feel the tightness, hold there and use your breath to deepen the stretch.

Keep your unextended hand on the thigh of your bent leg for support. When you feel comfortable, you can try extending both hands toward your flexed foot, as in the illustration. If that never happens for you, that's okay. People who are more flexible and can touch their toes with one hand will adjust to reaching with both hands equally in order to get the same stretch a beginner gets reaching with just one hand. Remember, you are only in competition with yourself!

15. Forward Bend

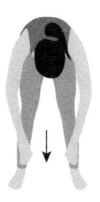

Do this movement slowly and gently. If standing, do not lock your knees. Your knees should be slightly bent, and you should not feel a stretch in the backs of your legs. This stretch is for your back.

➢ Stand or sit in alignment with your feet hip-width apart.

➢ Place your palms on your thighs.

➢ Slowly slide your palms down your legs.

➢ Follow your palms by bending at the waist.

➢ Remember to keep your knees slightly bent.

➢ When you get as far as you are going to go, your hands will leave your legs and dangle towards the floor. Let them do that. They'll know when.

➢ Allow the top of your head to dangle, too; it won't fall off!

➢ Shake your hands a little, breathe, and feel the gentle stretch all along your spine.

➢ Stay in this position as long as you like.

➢ When you are ready to stand, return your hands to your legs and slide them back up until you are standing.

➢ Once standing, gently roll your shoulders back and down to return them to their proper, aligned placement.

Ah, didn't that feel good?

16. Ankle Flexion

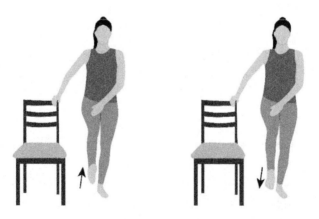

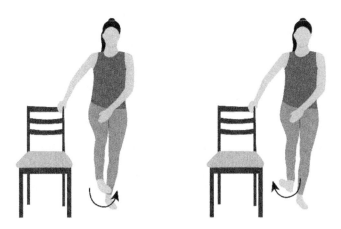

Do this exercise seated or standing. If standing, hold onto a chair for support. Remember to keep the knee of the leg you are standing on slightly bent because it gives you more support.

➢ Sit or stand in alignment.

➢ Lift one leg off of the floor, bending your knee at a 90° angle.

➢ Point your toe forward and then flex your foot for a count of 10 (1=point, 2=flex, etc.).

➢ Circle your foot outward 5 times.

➢ Circle your foot inward 5 times.

➢ Return your foot to the floor.

➢ Repeat on the other side.

Congratulations! You finished the warmup. This routine can take anywhere from 10 to 20 minutes depending on the amount of time you take with your deepening breaths. Deeper, longer breaths are more beneficial and take more time. It is possible to run through the warmup exercises in half the time if you perform them in a more superficial way. You will still be fully warmed up and ready for more.

Use this routine strictly as a warmup by foregoing taking full, deepening breaths.

Use this routine as a deep stretch by taking your time to deepen the stretches fully.

CHAPTER 3

The Workout—Core Exercises

A s I said in Chapter 1, the core is the base of the body's strength. Core strength is essential in developing muscle in the rest of the body. It helps to trim belly fat, too! According to the Mayo Clinic, core exercises "train the muscles in your pelvis, lower back, hips and abdomen to work in harmony. This leads to better balance and stability…" (Mayo Clinic Staff, 2017b). For any exercise to qualify as a core exercise, it just needs to involve the coordinated use of the muscles in the back and the abs. Not only will core exercises tone your abs, more importantly for seniors, they make it easier to do everyday activities, help improve posture, and reduce back pain.

Remember to complete the warmup in Chapter 2 before doing these exercises so that your body is prepared for more strenuous activity. Make sure you understand all instructions, and take it easy the first time through. You can add more reps and speed once you understand the movements. Remember that doing fewer exercises mindfully and completely will get you where you want to go faster than doing too much too quickly.

Routine 1: Seated Core Exercises

For these exercises, use a stable chair with a flat seat and no armrests.

1. **Spine Warmer**

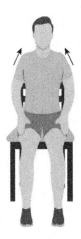 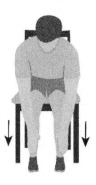

This is similar to the seated forward bend in the warmup routine. It is intended to engage both your back and your ab muscles. Imagine your movement originating in your core command center.

➤ Sit in alignment at the front of your chair with your feet flat on the floor and your hands on your thighs. Inhale.

➤ As you exhale, slowly slide your hands down your legs all the way to your ankles.

➤ As you inhale, slowly slide your hand back up.

➤ When you reach your seated position, roll your shoulders back and down.

➤ Repeat for a total of 4.

2. Ab Warmer

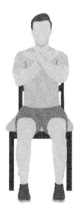 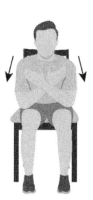

➤ Sit in alignment.

➤ Cross your arms over your chest like Dracula in his coffin. Inhale.

➢ As you exhale, bend forward until your elbows touch your knees.

➢ As you inhale, return to your upright, seated position.

➢ Repeat for a total of 4.

To increase the benefit of this exercise, press your belly button toward your spine as you bend forward and exhale.

3. **Bracing the Core**

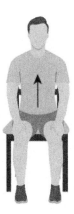

➢ Sit in alignment with your hands on your thighs. Really feel like you're sitting up nice and tall with your shoulders relaxed down.

➢ On an exhale, press your belly button toward your spine (suck in your gut).

➢ Hold for a slow count of 10.

➢ Relax and take a deep breath to replenish your oxygen.

➢ Breathe normally a couple of times.

➢ Repeat for a total of 4.

You can repeat this exercise up to four times once you are familiar with the routine. For the exercises throughout the book, **"brace your core"** means tighten your stomach muscles before and during any movement. It will feel like doing about half of the sucking in you just did. You should be able to breathe easily with your core braced.

4. Seated Side Bend

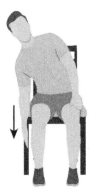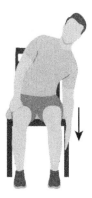

➢ Sit in alignment with your right hand on your right thigh and your left hand hanging toward the floor on your left side.

➢ Brace your core.

➢ Reach for the floor with your dangling hand. The hand on your thigh should remain on your thigh.

➢ When you get as far as you can go (you won't touch the floor, so don't expect to), sit back up.

➢ Lean down again immediately for a total of 5 reaches.

➢ After the fifth reach, sit up, release your core, and take a few recovery breaths.

➢ Repeat on the other side.

➢ Do each side twice.

This is not a side stretch. It is for your oblique abs. It is extremely important that your core is braced during the movement, or you won't get the intended benefit. The reason that you don't push your abs all the way to the back, as in the previous exercise, is that you need to be able to breathe while you move. If you fully suck in your gut, you cut off your ability to take in air. So, remember to breathe while you are moving.

5. **Leaning Back**

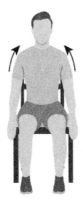 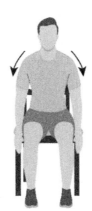

This is like a seated sit up. It is important to keep your aligned posture while you move. Think of Dracula again, sitting up in his coffin. His torso is perfectly straight and aligned, and yours should be, too. Bracing the core is the secret to success. This is an excellent exercise for solid core strength and will help if you have lower back problems.

> ➤ Sit in alignment at the front of your chair with your arms dangling at your sides.

> ➤ Brace your core.

> ➤ Slowly, hinge back as far as you can (you probably won't reach the back of the chair).

➢ When you've leaned back as far as you can while still maintaining your core brace and your aligned posture, hinge back up.

➢ Lean back and up 5 times.

➢ Release your core, rest, and breathe.

➢ Repeat.

Your feet should not come off the floor. Stop your movement back if this starts to happen because it means that that's as far as you can go and still maintain your aligned posture. With practice, you might be able to work up to leaning all the way to the back of the chair and still keep your feet on the floor. When you can do that, you'll be ready for the Olympics!

6. Seated We're Not Worthy!

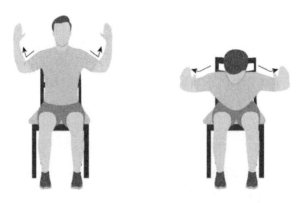

Ready to get your Wayne or Garth on?

➢ Sit in alignment at the front of the chair with your arms raised to the sides like you're under arrest.

➢ Brace your core.

➢ Bend all the way forward, keeping your head aligned with your spine so that when you have bent all the way forward, your eyes see the ground between your feet.

➢ Hinge back up, keeping your arms in the same position throughout.

➢ Hinge forward and back 5 times, keeping your core braced.

➢ Release your core, rest, and breathe.

➢ Repeat.

7. Seated Leg Lifts

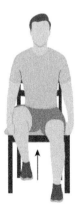
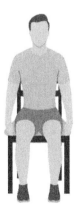

➤ Sit in alignment at the front of your chair and grip the seat with your hands.

➤ Brace your core.

➤ Lift and lower your right knee 5 times, making sure that the bottom of your foot makes full contact with the floor before you lift again.

➤ Repeat with your left knee.

➤ Rest.

➤ Repeat each side again.

This is a great exercise to practice moving from your core command center. Try it without doing that, and then try it by thinking of lifting your leg with your belly button. You should feel a difference—and get a better workout. Remember to keep your core braced the entire time you are moving.

As you get stronger, increase the number of times you raise your knee from five, to eight, to twelve.

8. **Heel and Toe Taps**

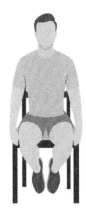 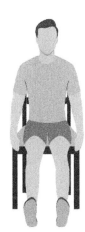

Sitting at the front of your chair for this is challenging if your abs aren't strong. The farther back on the seat you are, the easier this is. As your core gets stronger, move closer to the edge of your seat. Remember to maintain your aligned posture.

➤ Sit in alignment gripping the seat with your hands.

➤ Brace your core.

➤ Extend your legs and tap your heels on the floor.

➤ Bend your knees and tap your toes on the floor just under your chair.

➤ Count 10 (1=heel tap, 2=toe tap, and so on).

➤ Rest and repeat.

9. **Bicycle**

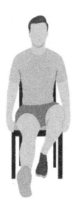 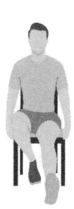

Ready to ride your bicycle where you like? Great! Remember to brace your core and initiate movement from your core command center. If you feel the exercise in your legs more than in your abs, you do not have your core properly braced. Imagining your belly button boss in charge can correct that.

> ➤ Sit in alignment at the front of your chair and grip the seat with your hands.

> ➤ Brace your core.

> ➤ Keeping your straight alignment, lean back just enough to raise your legs and "pedal" your bicycle forward for a count of 20.

> ➤ Return to your aligned seated posture and rest.

➢ Repeat but this time pedal your bicycle backward for a count of 20.

If 20 is too much, try for 12 and work your way up. Your abs should be feeling nice and warm and tingly by now. And hey, maybe they're saying it's time to stop. Hang in there—we're at the cool down

10. **Spine Relaxer**

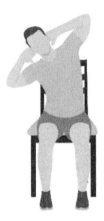 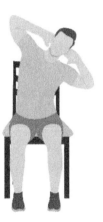

For this exercise, you need only brace your core at 25%— just enough to support the movement but not enough to continue seriously working the abs.

➢ Sit in alignment at the front of your chair and rest your hands behind your head.

➢ Lightly engage your core.

➢ Using your hands to support your head and prevent it from moving, slowly and gently lean to the right and then to the left for a count of 8 (four bends to each side). Think of it as lowering your elbow toward the floor.

Your goal is to release any tension built up in the spine during the core work. If you hear any pops or cracks, that is the sound of tension releasing.

11. **Recovery Stretch**

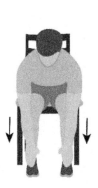
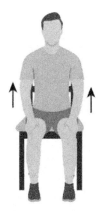

➢ Sit in alignment with your palms on your thighs and your legs extended in front of you, heels on the floor. Inhale.

➢ As you exhale, slide your palms down your legs to your ankles.

➢ As you inhale, slide your palms back up to your thighs.

➢ Once you return to sitting, roll your shoulders back and down.

➢ Repeat.

➢ Take a couple of deep breaths and let them go.

➢ Return to seated alignment with your feet flat on the floor. Inhale.

➢ Place your hands lightly behind your head for support.

➢ As you exhale, gently arch your back toward the back of the chair.

➢ Return to aligned posture, keeping your hands where they are. Inhale.

➢ As you exhale, stretch your arms up over your head.

➢ Get as much of a stretch as you want and then fly your arms back down to the sides and place them on your thighs.

➢ Take one last, deep relaxing breath and...you're done!

Routine 2: Mat Core Exercises

Mat exercises require you to get down on the floor. If you have serious lower back problems that make this difficult, like degenerative disc disease or arthritis, work with the chair exercises first. Then, you can add the mat exercises when you are stronger.

Lying on your back can cause pain for people with lower back problems. If this is you, and you do get down on the floor, keeping your knees bent and your feet flat on the floor will alleviate most of the pain or discomfort in your lower back.

Resting position for these exercises requires lying on your back and hugging your knees to your chest. This position should alleviate all pressure on your lower spine and fully rest your abs.

Do these exercises on a yoga mat, area rug, or any carpeted floor. I don't recommend that you do them on a bare wood or tile floor. You can also do them lying on a firm mattress.

Getting safely down to the floor

- ➢ Using a chair back for support, lower first one knee and then the other to the floor.

- ➢ Place your hands on the floor and turn yourself around so that you are sitting on your bottom. Your legs can be crossed or extended—it doesn't matter so long as it's comfortable for you.

➤ Place your hands on the floor just behind your hips with your fingers pointing toward your feet and slowly lower yourself down onto your elbows.

➤ Once you are on your elbows, put your feet flat on the floor with your knees pointing toward the ceiling.

➤ Lower yourself onto your back.

➤ Adjust your position as needed for maximum comfort.

Getting safely up off the floor

➤ Roll onto one side.

➤ Use your hands to push yourself up to sitting.

➤ Once you are sitting, come to your hands and knees.

➤ Using your hands to balance, get your feet onto the floor underneath you.

➤ Push against the floor to begin to rise.

➤ Shift your hands to your thighs and push against them to get all the way up.

This routine is not recommended for beginners or those with low physical strength. *However, if you have no problem getting up and down from the floor, you should be able to handle it. Just remember to listen to your body as* *you slowly go through it the first time. If you experience any pain or too much difficulty, stop and use the Seated Core Exercises instead. Remember to complete the warmup before doing either routine.*

Lie comfortably on your back *means with your feet flat on the floor, your knees pointing toward the ceiling, and your palms flat on the floor next to your hips.*

1. Reverse Crunch

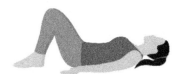 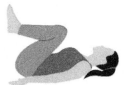

Let's work your lower abs. Initiate the movement from your core command center instead of from your legs.

- ➢ Lie comfortably on your back. Inhale.

- ➢ As you exhale, press your belly button toward your spine and lift your feet off the floor, bringing your knees toward your chest.

- ➢ Once they are as far up as they will go, hold them there for a count of two. Inhale as you hold.

➢ Exhale, push your belly button toward your spine, and lower your feet back to the floor.

➢ Repeat for a total of 5.

If it is too difficult for you to raise both legs together, you can raise them separately. Alternate right and left for a count of 10 (five on each side). When you are stronger, you will be able to do both legs together.

2. Gentle Knee Drops to the Side

Lie comfortably on your back. Slowly, allow your knees to move to the right until they want to stop; then, move them to the left. Swing them slowly left and right for a count of 8 (four times on each side). Breathe normally while doing this. This is a recovery move that provides your spine with a slight twist that opens up your lower vertebrae.

3. Upper Ab Squeeze

Because traditional crunches can be dangerous for anyone when done improperly, and especially for seniors and people with neck problems, we replace them with this exercise that gives the same benefit without the danger of strain or injury.

➢ Lie comfortably on your back. Inhale.

➢ As you exhale, squeeze your ab muscles as tight as you can.

➢ Hold for a count of eight with no breath.

➢ Release and take a few recovery breaths.

➤ Repeat for a total of 4 squeezes.

You will not be able to breathe while you squeeze. If you cannot hold for a count of 8, start with a count of 4, then 6, then build up to 8.

This is not the same as "sucking in your gut." You want to tense all of your ab muscles at once. Try doing both to feel the difference so that you can know you are doing it correctly.

Recover *in Resting Position, feet off the floor and knees up toward your chest.*

4. Modified Tuck Crunch

➤ Lie comfortably on your back, hands behind your head. Inhale.

➤ As you exhale, squeeze your abs and lift your feet off the floor, bringing your knees toward your chest. Do NOT hold.

➤ Exhale and return your feet to the floor.

➢ Repeat for a total of 5.

As with the Reverse Crunch, you can alternate legs at first if you need to.

Recover *with Gentle Knee Drops to the Side or Resting Position.*

5. **Reverse Table Top Extensions**

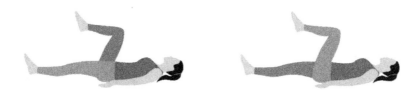

Starting position for this exercise is important. Use the illustration as a guide. This should feel comfortable and not present any type of strain.

➢ Lie comfortably on your back and bring your feet off the floor, knees at 90°.

➢ Softly flex your feet so that your toes point toward the ceiling. Inhale.

➢ As you exhale, keep your foot flexed, extend your right leg toward the floor, and then bring it back to starting position. Inhale.

➢ Repeat with your other leg.

➤ Repeat for a count of 10 (five extensions on each leg).

Remember to initiate the movement from your core command center instead of from your leg. This not only works your core, it also prevents strain on your lower back and makes the extension easier.

Don't touch the floor with your heel. Extend the leg so that your heel is one to two inches from the floor and then pull it back.

This exercise not only strengthens your core, but works your thigh muscles and hip flexors too!

Recover *with Gentle Knee Drops to the Side or Resting Position. Modify Gentle Knee Drops by crossing one leg over the other before initiating the rocking motion. Then, reverse your cross and do the drops again. This will give you a deeper spinal stretch than doing it with both feet flat on the floor.*

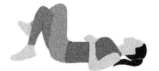 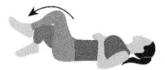

6. **Reverse Leg and Arm Extensions**

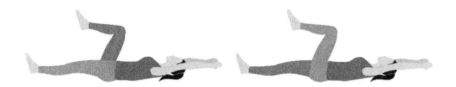

Add arm motions to Table Top Extension for a greater challenge. Don't forget to brace your core before you start the extension movements.

> ➢ Lie comfortably on your back and bring your feet off the floor, knees at 90°, feet flexed.

> ➢ Raise your arms straight up from your chest, fingers toward the ceiling. Inhale.

> ➢ As you exhale, extend your right leg, keeping your foot flexed, and extend both arms over your head. Bring leg and arms back to starting position. Inhale.

> ➢ Repeat with your other leg.

> ➢ Repeat for a count of 10 (five extensions on each leg).

Recover *with Resting Position.*

7. Table Top Extensions

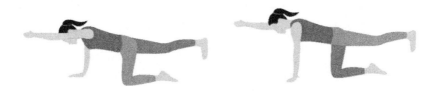

This is a classic yoga core and balance exercise that strengthens the lower back. It should be done on the floor. If you have knee problems, use knee pads or put extra padding under your knees, like a folded blanket or soft towel.

Starting position is extremely important for balance. Begin on your hands and knees. Notice that in the illustration, the knee is directly beneath the hip, and the hand is directly beneath the shoulder. The back is flat, and the top of the head is pointed toward the wall, not dropped. When both hands and both knees are on the floor, you should form an almost perfect square with your torso, arms, and thighs.

> ➢ Come into Table Top position. Inhale.

> ➢ As you exhale, engage your core command center and extend your right leg back and your left arm forward at the same time.

> ➢ Balance in this position as you inhale. Exhale. Inhale.

➢ As you exhale, return to starting position.

➢ Repeat on the other side.

➢ Alternate sides for a total of 4 extensions on each side.

If you need additional support while holding the pose, you can put a chair behind you and rest the top of your extended foot on the seat while you breathe.

If four extensions on each side is too much at first, start with one or two and work your way up.

8. **Belly Extension**

This exercise works your lower back as well as your core. It is a bit more difficult than Table Top Extensions, so take it slowly. It is not necessary to lift your leg or arm a foot off the floor as shown in the illustration, if this is too difficult. A couple of inches is fine. As always, do what you can, and you can work up to more.

➢ Lower yourself onto your belly from Table Top position. Inhale.

➢ As you exhale, lift your right leg and your left arm off the floor at the same time.

➢ As you inhale, lower your leg and arm. Do not hold.

➢ On your next exhale, lift your left leg and your right arm.

➢ Lower them as you inhale.

➢ Continue on alternate sides for a count of 8 (four on each side).

Ideally, you are working with each breath. Up on the exhale and down on the inhale; then, up on the other side as you exhale again. If this pace is too much, you can take a recovery breath between each lift.

9. **Cat (but maybe not) Cow**

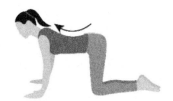 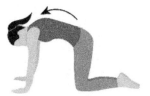

This final exercise is good for both abs and spine, however, I don't recommend "Cow" for seniors with lower back problems. If you attempt Cow and experience any pain or discomfort beyond what you would describe as mild, simply return to Table Top position before your next Cat.

> ➢ Begin in Table Top position. Inhale.

> ➢ As you exhale, lower your head between your arms, press your belly button to your spine, and arch your back like an angry Halloween cat. Pushing against the floor with your hands will help you get a higher arch. Exhale fully.

> ➢ As you inhale, return to Table Top position.

> ➢ Take a recovery breath.

> ➢ Repeat for a total of 5.

If you want to attempt Cow, instead of stopping in Table Top position on your inhale, let your belly continue to sink toward the floor. Your head should come up so that you are looking at the wall instead of the floor, and your spine will arch in the opposite direction, downward. Return to Table Top position for a recovery breath before going on to your next Cat.

If you feel any pain trying to do Cow, don't do it. Cat works your abs and back. Cow allows for deeper relaxation in your spine. However, if you feel pain or discomfort instead of relaxation, Cow is not something you need to do.

10. **Recover with Child's Pose.**

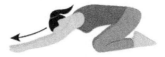

> From Table Top position, bring your feet together and spread your knees wide.

> Push against the floor with your hands, sending your bottom back toward your feet. Stop when it gets as far as it is going to go.

> Slowly slide your hands forward until your forearms meet the floor.

> Rest your forehead and your forearms on the floor and breathe deeply into your belly.

This is a resting pose. Once you are in it, you should feel relaxed. Stay here for as much or as little time as you want—you're done!

Routine 3: Belly Fat Exercises

This short, low-impact aerobics routine elevates your heart rate and burns belly fat. I suggest putting on some fun, upbeat music you really love, and get ready to move to the music! Wear sturdy athletic shoes that provide support and traction.

1. **March in Place**

March in place for a few measures just to warm up a little and get into the groove.

2. **Twist and Lift**

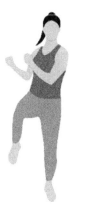
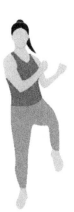

➢ Stand with your feet hip-width apart and your hands held up before you like a champion boxer.

➢ Turn your torso right, left, right, left to get the feel of the movement. Don't turn all the way to the side (15 on a clock). Only turn as far as you can remain relaxed and comfortable (about 7 on a clock).

➢ Count up from one, and on three lift your heel but leave your toe on the floor: 1=rotate right, 2=rotate left, 3=rotate right and lift your right heel.

➢ Continue with the movement, starting over at one, and the next time, you will lift your left heel.

➢ Continue for at least 30 seconds. You can easily gauge this by counting: 1-2-3, 2-2-3, 3-2-3, and so on up to 10-2-3.

➢ Repeat, but this time lift your foot on three instead of just lifting your heel.

➢ Repeat, but this time lift your knee.

Shift your weight as you rotate to accommodate lifting your foot or leg. If you find that you are off balance, you probably aren't shifting your weight. Your heart rate should be slightly elevated but not pounding. If it is a little faster than your resting heart rate, you are burning fat! If your heart is pounding, slow down and do less.

3. **Mountain Climber**

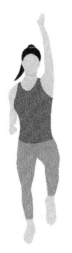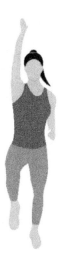

> ➤ Stand with your feet directly beneath your hips.

> ➤ Raise those boxer's fists again, but lift them up above your head.

> ➤ Lift your right heel off the floor as you pull your right fist down toward your chest.

> ➤ Set your right heel down as you punch up toward the ceiling with your fist.

> ➤ Repeat on the left side.

> ➤ Practice that a couple of times, and then do both at once, meaning: lift your left heel off the floor as you pull your left fist down and, at the same time, thrust your right fist back up over your head and set your right heel down.

➢ Continue for a count of 30. (If that's too much, start with ten).

➢ Repeat, but this time lift your right knee in a march step instead of just lifting your heel. This time you will feel more like the leader of a marching band with a baton in each hand.

➢ Continue for a count of 30.

Doing the hand-and-foot coordination this way (right hand and right foot moving together) will help your balance.

Challenge your balance: lift the left foot as you pull down the right fist. This is more difficult, but excellent for balance. I recommend mastering same-side first and then moving on to opposite-side coordination.

Modification: if having your arms extended over your head is too much at first, start with your fists thrust out in front of your chest, and pull back toward your chest as you lift your heel or leg. You can also switch back and forth, punching at the ceiling until you get tired, then punching out in front of you for a bit of a rest as you continue your footwork, and then returning to punching toward the ceiling when you're ready.

4. **Step and Push**

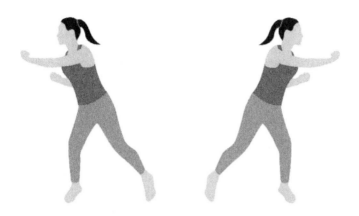

➢ Stand with your feet below your hips and your boxer fists raised at your chest.

➢ Take a comfortable step to the right with your right foot.

➢ Close that space by bringing your left over next to your right foot.

➢ Take a second step to the right, but turn your right foot like you are going to walk in that direction.

➢ Allow your left foot to pivot to accommodate that movement.

➢ As you turn to face the right, push your left palm across your body toward the right.

➤ Bend your right knee for support and tap your left toe as you complete the push.

➤ As you bring your left hand back to your chest, turn your body so that you face front (where your started)

➤ Close the space between your feet by bringing your right foot next to your left foot.

➤ Step out to the left like you are going to walk that way, your right foot pivoting to allow the movement, and push your right hand across your body to the left.

➤ As you complete the push, bend your left knee for support, and tap your right toe.

➤ As you bring your right hand back to your chest, return to facing front.

➤ Continue in this manner, counting each time you push a hand up to 30 (fifteen pushes on each side).

The illustration shows the back foot raised on the toe—that is that back foot tapping.

This exercise is easier than the previous one and provides a bit of a cool down while still maintaining your elevated heart rate. Again, if your heart starts pounding, you are doing too much, and the exercise is no longer benefiting your cardiovascular health. Slow down.

5. Starfish

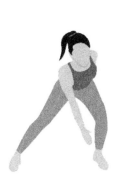 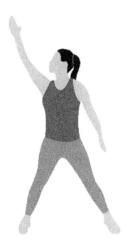

This will bring your heart rate up and strengthen your thighs. Do what you can and listen to your heart.

➢ Stand with your feet wide and bend one your right knee. Keep your right hand resting on your upper thigh for balance.

➢ Reach toward your ankle with your left hand. Don't try to touch your toes—about mid-calf level is perfect (see illustration).

➢ This is your starting place.

➢ From this position, straighten your bent knee and swing your arm up to a capital Y position.

➢ Swing your arm down, bend your knee, and return to starting position.

➢ Straighten your bent knee and swing your arm out to the side, parallel to the floor.

➢ Return to starting position.

➢ Count 12 (six each for the Y position and parallel position).

➢ Repeat on the other side.

Keep moving once you start—it should flow. Use your music.

The figure in the illustration does not have a hand on the thigh. Once you have mastered the exercise using the support of your hand on your thigh, you can remove it for a greater challenge.

Challenge modification: bring your bent leg over to meet your standing leg as you complete the parallel arm movement and then move it back as you return to starting position.

6. **Patty Cake Protection**

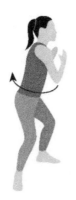
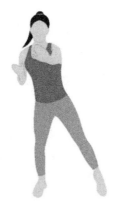

➢ Stand with your feet hip width apart and palms together before your chest.

➢ With your right foot, step out to the right and back. Turn to the right, bend your knees, and sink your body like a ninja ready for action. You now face right.

➢ As you turn out, separate your palms and bring your fists into boxer mode.

➢ Push off with your right foot and return to stand facing forward. Clap once.

➢ Extend your left foot back to tap your toe, and patty-cake your left hand all the way out across your body.

➢ Return to front and clap once.

➢ Repeat the movement to the other side: extend your right foot back to tap your toe, and patty-cake your right hand all the way across your body.

➢ Return to starting position with your palms together.

➢ Repeat on the other side: step out to the left and back. Turn left, bend your knees, sink your body like a ninja, and look for enemies with your fists raised.

➢ Return to front and continue to patty cake in safety. First right, then left.

➢ Repeat for a total of 12 (six on each side).

Feel how solid and grounded you are in your ninja crouch. If you don't feel stable, bend your knees more so that you feel like a tiger ready to spring.

This is also good for thinking and coordination. Here is the sequence in case you are confused. PC stands for Patty Cake. First set—ninja right, PC left, PC right. Second set—ninja left, PC right, PC left.

Challenge modification – the lower you crouch the more you work your thighs and increase cardio.

Cool Down by dancing to that funky music you put on for a minute.

Getting through this routine once with some peppy music (once you get the hang of the exercises) should take about ten minutes. If you want a longer workout, you can repeat the sequence or increase the number of repetitions of each exercise the first time through.

There are three complete routines in this chapter. Try them all and then cycle through them as you build your personal, weekly exercise plan.

CHAPTER 4

The Workout—Arms and Shoulders

I t can be difficult not having the strength you used to take for granted. Upper body strength training has several benefits for seniors including positively affecting cognitive function, combating osteoporosis, increasing the mineral content of bones, and reversing muscle loss due to the aging process (Pain Relief Institute, 2019).

These exercises are focused directly on the arms and shoulders and not on the core, but remember that the more you engage your core, no matter what exercise you are performing, the greater the benefits will be and the faster they will occur.

Routine 1: Seated Arm Strength

Don't forget to do your warmup first. As you work through the routine, feel free to shake out your arms between exercises to give them a little rest and release tension. Ready? Then, grab that sturdy chair and let's get started!

1. **Arm Curls**

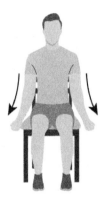 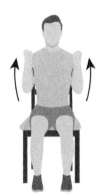

➤ Sit in alignment at the front of your chair with your feet flat on the floor.

➤ Extend your arms down at your sides with your fists closed, curled fingers facing front. Brace your core.

➤ Bend your elbows, bringing your fists toward your shoulders.

- ➤ Once there, give a little extra squeeze, really pushing your lower arm into your upper arm.

- ➤ Slowly lower your fists to your sides.

- ➤ Repeat 10 times, keeping your core braced.

Get maximum benefit by bracing your core and remembering to do that extra little squeeze before lowering your fists.

2. **Triceps Squeeze #1**

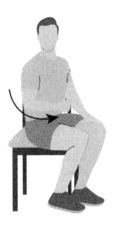
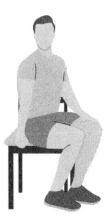

- ➤ Turn to the side on your chair and sit in alignment.

- ➤ Hold your closed fist at your side, like you have a beer, with your fingers facing in toward your body. Brace your core.

- ➤ Lower your fist toward the floor.

➢ When it gets there, give it an extra little squeeze so that you feel the muscle in the back of your arm flex.

➢ Raise your fist to starting position.

➢ Repeat 10 times on each side, keeping your core braced.

3. Triceps Squeeze #2

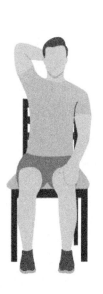 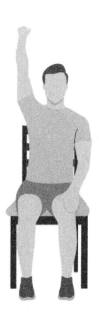

➢ Sit in alignment facing front.

➢ Rest one hand on your thigh. Raise and bend your other arm so that your fist is behind your head, and your elbow points out to the side. Brace your core.

➢ Raise your fist over your head.

- ➢ At the top, give that extra little squeeze to work that tricep.

- ➢ Slowly lower your arm to starting position.

- ➢ Repeat 10 times on each side, keeping your core braced.

Ladies (and some gentlemen), a ponytail or bun is going to get in the way of doing this correctly, so be prepared to take it down.

Make sure your elbow is angled out toward the side and not angling in toward the front for maximum benefit.

4. **Easy Shoulder Rotation**

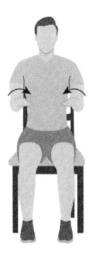 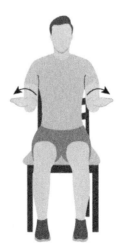

➢ Sit in alignment facing forward.

➢ Raise your Frankenstein arms with your palms open.

➢ Breathe easily as you gently rotate your hands so that your palms face up.

➢ Continue rotating up and down for 10, counting each time your palms turn up.

The more you extend your arms, the more you engage your shoulders.

5. **Wrist Flexion**

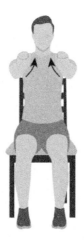
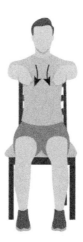

➢ Remember to maintain good posture and alignment as you sit.

➢ Extend your arms in front of you with your fists closed like you're on a motorcycle.

➤ Breathe easily as you gently flex your wrists so that your knuckles point toward the ceiling.

➤ Reverse so that your knuckles point toward the floor.

➤ Continue flexing up and down for 10, counting each time you flex upward.

If it is difficult for you to hold your arms out in front of you for this exercise, you can let your arms hang at your sides while you flex your wrists.

6. **Triceps Extensions**

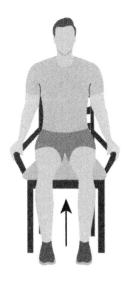 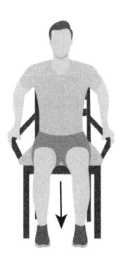

You will need a chair with sturdy armrests for this exercise.

➢ Sit in alignment in the chair and place your hands on the armrests. Inhale.

➢ As you exhale, brace your core and push against the armrests to raise yourself in the chair.

➢ Hold for the length of your exhale.

➢ Inhale, release and relax.

➢ Repeat 10 times.

Don't use your legs to help raise your body. Use the weight of your body to strengthen your arm muscles. You don't have to raise your bottom off the seat. Press until you feel your arms working and hold it there until you finish your exhale. Over time, you will be able to lift yourself higher.

If you like, you can add weights to these exercises. If you do, follow the instructions as written, always including that extra little squeeze.

Routine 2: Standing Arm Toner

Complete your warmup before this routine. If you need to drop your arms before you finish with an exercise, try to go two movements more than you think you can before you relax. Remember to initiate the arm movements from your core command center and work with your core braced. Doing so will not only strengthen your core as you strengthen your arms, it will also give you more stamina for the arm movements. Put some fun music on, too!

1. **Lateral Arm Raises**

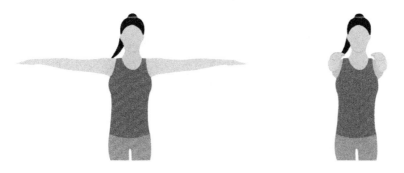

- ➢ Stand in alignment with your palms just touching the outer fronts of your thighs.

- ➢ Raise and extend your arms in front of you at chest level with your palms facing the floor.

- ➢ Swing your arms out to the sides like you are making a "t".

- ➢ Swing your arms back in front of you.

- ➢ Lower your arms back to where they started.

- ➢ Repeat: raise, swing out, swing in, lower for 15, counting one each time you raise your arms in front of you. Or if you want to use a timer, set it for 60 seconds.

2. **Back Pulses**

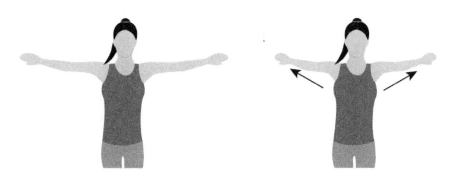

➢ Stand in alignment and raise your arms out to the sides with your palms facing behind you.

➢ Imagine that there is something just behind you that you need to push back.

➢ Gently pulse your arms back for a count of 60 (one minute).

You can use a timer, but you will probably do one pulse per second, so counting to sixty will get you to a minute. If that's too much, that's okay. Just do two more pulses than you think you can, and then stop. You can build up to 60.

3. **Front Pulses**

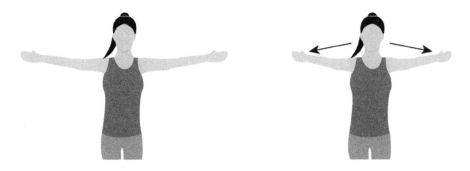

➢ Raise your arms as in Back Pulses but face your palms forward.

➢ Imagine that there is something you have to push forward in front of you.

➢ Gently pulse your arms forward for a count of 60.

4. **Scoops**

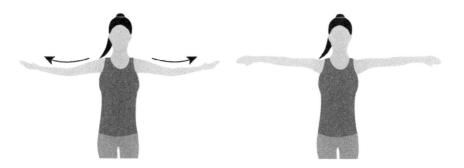

➢ Raise your arms out to the sides with your palms facing up but your hands cupped like you want to catch some raindrops.

➢ Rotate your hands forward and all the way around until your cupped hands are facing the wall behind you.

➢ Rotate back to starting position.

➢ Imagine that you are scooping sand or water in your hand and pushing it back behind you and then returning for more.

➢ Repeat for one minute (or a count of 25).

5. **Taps**

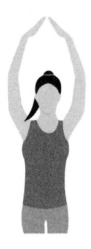 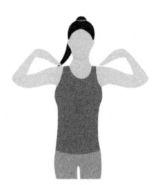

➢ Stand in alignment with your arms extended to the sides, palms up.

➢ Bend your elbows and tap your shoulders.

➢ Return to starting position.

➢ Raise your arms and tap your fingertips together overhead.

➢ Return to starting position.

➢ You have completed one set.

➢ Repeat for one minute (or a count of 18 sets)

6. Step Off, I'm Hiding

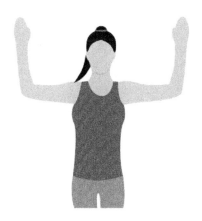 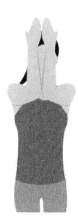

➢ Stand in alignment with your arms extended to the sides and your elbows bent at a right angle.

➢ Bring your arms together, turning your palms toward your face for "I'm Hiding."

➢ Swing your arms back out to your sides.

➢ When they are open (as shown in the illustration), turn your palms outward and give a tiny push for "Step Off."

➢ Alternate between the two for one minute (or a count of 20 pairs).

You could just return your arms to the starting position after hiding, but that extra little twist and push makes this exercise doubly effective.

7. **Powerful Arm Raises**

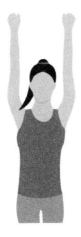 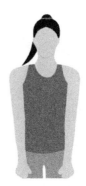

- ➢ Stand in alignment with your arms hanging down in front of you and your hands in fists.

- ➢ Raise your fists straight out in front of you. Pause.

- ➢ Raise your fists up over your head. Pause.

- ➢ Lower your fists back to straight out in front of you.

- ➢ Swing your fists out to the sides.

- ➢ Swing your fists back to straight out in front of you.

- ➢ Lower your fists back to starting position.

- ➢ Repeat the series for one minute (or 10 ten sets, counting each time your arms raise overhead).

8. Shoulder Taps

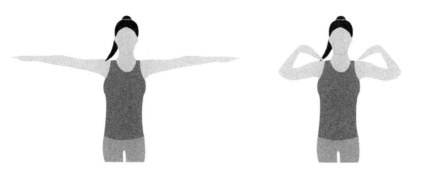

➤ Stand in alignment with your arms extended out to the sides, palms up.

➤ Bend your elbows and tap your shoulders.

➤ Return to starting position.

➤ Repeat for one minute (or 25 taps).

9. Crosses

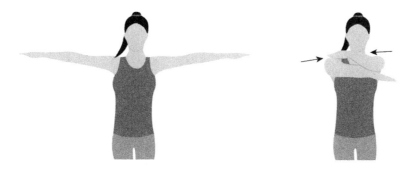

➢ Stand in alignment with your arms extended out to the sides, palms down.

➢ With your arms extended, cross them in front of you, right over left. Don't bend your elbows; keep your arms straight.

➢ Return to starting position.

➢ Cross your arms again, this time left over right.

➢ Continue crossing and alternating the arm that is above for one minute (or 25 crosses).

10. **Arm Circles, Palms Down**

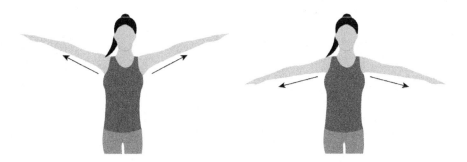

➢ Stand in alignment with your arms extended out to the sides, palms down.

➢ Slowly circle your arms forward.

➢ Imagine that your extended fingers are tracing the outline of a dinner plate; your arm circles don't need to be any bigger than that.

➢ Continue for one minute (or 40 circles).

Cool down by stretching your arms over her head, or shaking them out, or both.

Routine 3: Seated Shoulder Strength #1

Since these exercises target the shoulders, it is important to keep your shoulders relaxed down while doing them. Remember that it's impossible to keep your shoulders relaxed if your head is not in the proper position, so pull up on those ears.

1. **Graduated Shoulder Flexion**

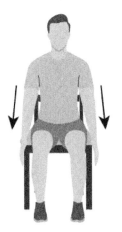
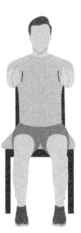

Shoulder flexion is movement that takes your arms from your sides up over your head. This exercise brings you there gradually.

➤ Sit in alignment at the front of your chair, hands hanging at your sides, palms facing in toward each other. Brace your core.

➤ Gently raise your arms straight out in front of you.

➤ Lower your arms slowly.

➤ Repeat for a total of 5.

➤ Release your core and take a few recovery breaths. When you are ready to lift your arms higher, brace your core.

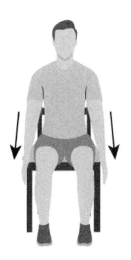 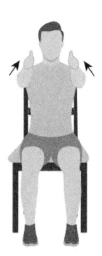

➤ Gently raise your arms just above shoulder level.

➤ Lower your arms, slow and controlled.

➤ Repeat for a total of 5.

➢ Release your core and take a few recovery breaths. When you are ready to lift your arms over your head, brace your core.

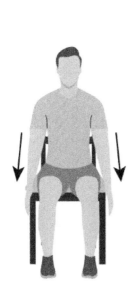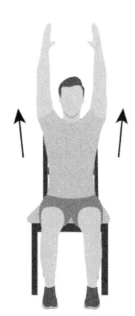

➢ Gently raise your arms up over your head.

➢ Slowly lower your arms all the way down.

➢ Repeat for a total of 10.

➢ When you have your arms overhead the tenth time, pause and release your core.

➢ Stretch up toward the ceiling with your right hand. Relax that side.

➢ Stretch up toward the ceiling with your left hand. Relax that side.

➢ Slowly, return both arms to your sides and give them a gentle shake.

If you can't raise your arms all the way up, that's okay. Go as far as you comfortably can and come back down. Your range of motion will improve as you do this exercise over time.

Control your movement up and down — slow and steady. Not allowing your arms to relax when they come back down will help strengthen the muscles in your arms as well as increase the range of motion in your shoulders—two for one!

2. **Shoulder Press**

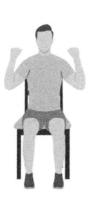 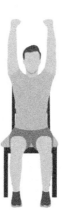

As with the previous exercise, if your arms are not ready to go all the way up, don't force them.

➢ Sit in alignment at the front of your chair with your arms raised out the sides and your fists facing front.

Imagine that you are holding onto a bar that sits on your shoulders, like a milkmaid. Inhale.

➤ As you exhale, press your belly button to your spine and raise up over your head.

➤ Lower all the way down to starting position on your inhale.

➤ Repeat for a total of 10.

Abs go in and arms go up—use your breath!

Recover by shaking out your arms and taking a couple of nice, long breaths.

3. **Bent Elbow Arm Swings**

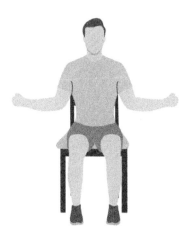 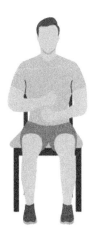

The trick to this exercise is to keep your elbows close to your sides. As you swing your arms out, your elbows will naturally come away from your sides. You are on a mission to make sure they stay as close as possible. As you do the exercise for the first time, notice the difference in muscle use if you insist that they remain close rather than allowing them to move away.

> ➢ Sit in alignment at the front of your chair with your elbows hugging your sides and your fists resting on your belly.

> ➢ As you exhale, engage your core and rotate your forearms open as far as they will go.

> ➢ When they get there, squeeze your elbows into your sides and release.

> ➢ As you inhale, rotate your forearms back to starting position and relax your core.

> ➢ Repeat for a total of 10.

> ➢ Recover as above.

4. **Graduated Side Flexion**

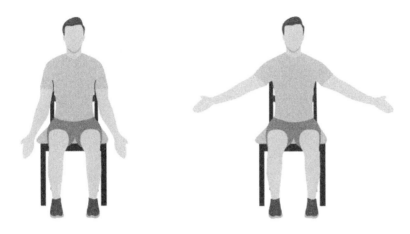

Again, only take your arms up as far as they can comfortably go on the final set of 10.

➢ Sit in alignment at the front of your chair with your arms hanging at your sides and your palms facing front. Brace your core.

➢ Raise your arms up 40° and lower them again, slow and controlled.

➢ Repeat for a total of 5.

➢ Release your core, take a couple of recovery breaths and get ready to lift your arms to shoulder height. When you're ready, brace your core.

➢ Raise and lower your arms to shoulder height. Control!

➢ Repeat for a total of 5.

➢ Release, recover, and prepare to raise your arms overhead. Ready? Brace your core.

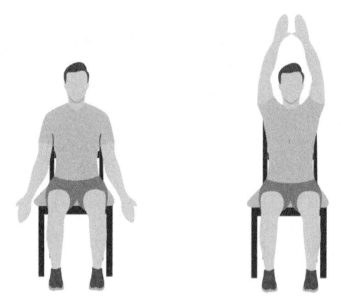

➢ Raise and lower your arms up over your head.

➢ Repeat for a total of 10, taking a moment to rest after 5.

Recover by shaking out your arms and taking a couple of deep breaths.

5. **Falcon**

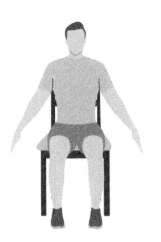 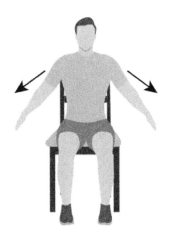

➢ Sit in alignment at the front of your chair with your arms extended down at our sides and your palms facing in. Check to make sure your shoulders are relaxed down.

➢ As you exhale, push your belly button to your spine, move your arms back, and press your shoulder blades together. Bring your arms back and up as far as you can without raising your shoulders.

➢ As you inhale, move your arms forward to starting position and relax your core.

➢ Repeat for a total of 10, taking a brief rest after 5.

6. Cool Down with Shoulder Rolls

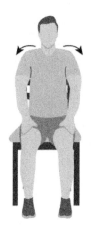 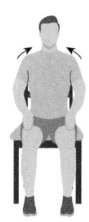

- ➢ Sit in alignment at the front of your chair with your palms resting on your knees.

- ➢ Breathe easily as you gently roll your shoulders back and all the way around for a count of 5.

- ➢ Allow your hands to move on your thighs as they follow the motion of your shoulders. And...

- ➢ You're done!

As you continue exploring and then using the various workouts, remember that building range of motion and strength will help you with everyday tasks like laundry, putting away groceries, and taking out the trash.

Routine 4: Seated Shoulder Strength #2

All rules apply—maintain posture, use your breath, engage your core, and be mindful that your shoulders stay relaxed down (or return there immediately after effort). You can do the routine seated or standing.

1. **Shoulder Blade Squeeze**

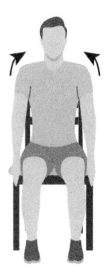 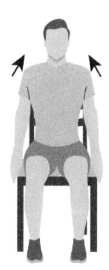

Remember this exercise from the warmup? Really allow your shoulders to relax each time you come down before you send them back up.

➢ Sit or stand in alignment.

➢ Lift your shoulders up toward your ears as you inhale. UP.

➢ Move your arms back and press your shoulder blades together as you exhale. BACK.

➢ Allow your shoulders to relax down as you finish exhaling. DOWN.

➢ Repeat for a total of 8.

2. **Graduated Arm Circles**

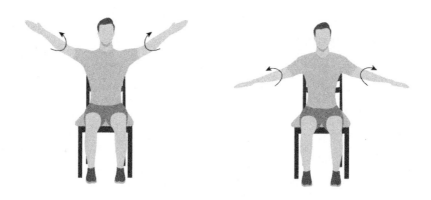

Work with your arms raised to shoulder height. If that is too hard or painful, you can lower your arms a little and still get the benefit. Remember to keep your head in place and your shoulders relaxed down while you circle your arms.

➢ Sit or stand in alignment with your arms raised out to your sides at shoulder height.

➢ Breathing easily, circle your arms forward in a small circle, about the size of a coaster, for a count of 10.

➢ Increase the size of the circle to about a saucer for a count of 10.

➢ Increase the size of the circle to a dinner plate for a count of 10.

➢ Don't let your shoulders creep up.

➢ Increase the size of the circle to a hula-hoop for a count of 10.

➢ Lower your arms, shake them out, and recover.

➢ Repeat but circle your arms back this time.

3. **Bent Elbow Arm Swings**

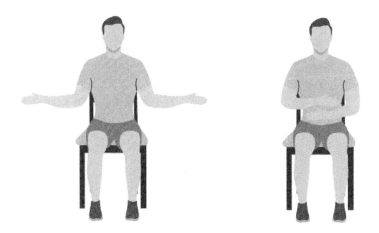

Keep your elbows close to your sides. For a greater challenge, hold a water bottle in each hand to add a little weight.

- ➤ Sit or stand in alignment with your elbows hugging your sides and your palms resting on your belly. Inhale.

- ➤ As you exhale, brace your core and rotate your forearms open as far as they will go.

- ➤ When they get there, squeeze your elbows into your sides and release.

- ➤ As you inhale, rotate your forearms back to starting position and relax your core.

- ➤ Repeat for a total of 10.

4. **Upward Rows**

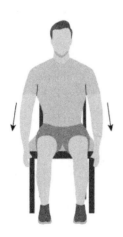 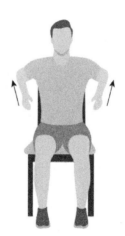

- ➤ Sit or stand in alignment with your fists at your sides. Brace your core.

➢ Raise your elbows behind you. Aim them at the ceiling and try to touch it with them.

➢ Be mindful and keep your shoulders relaxed down.

➢ Return your fists to starting position.

➢ Check to make sure your shoulders are relaxed before lifting them again.

➢ Repeat for a total of 10. Rest your core after 5.

5. **Up and Out**

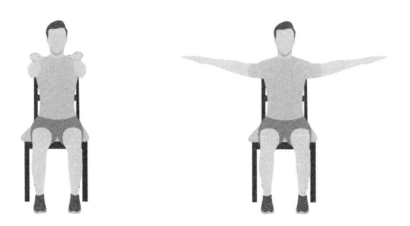

➢ Sit or stand in alignment with your arms hanging down.

➢ Breath easily as you lift your arms straight out in front of you and then lower them back to where they started.

➤ Keep breathing as you lift your arms out to the sides to shoulder height and lower them again.

➤ That was one set.

➤ Repeat for a total of 10 sets.

Keep the movement slow and easy. This is a bit of a cool down after the work of the first three exercises. As always, raise your arms only as high as you can with no pain. You will get the same benefit.

CHAPTER 5

The Workout—Legs and Hips

L eg and hip strength and flexibility are essential for our capacity to move around, to do for ourselves and for others, and to maintain independence. Those with lower back problems know the pain and frustration of a flare up that leaves them barely able to get out of bed or shuffle to the bathroom. Supple and strong muscles can help aid us during those times when inflammation seeks to cripple us. The rest of the time, having strong legs and flexible hips gives us more stamina for longer walks through the park or grocery store and other activities we either enjoy or are required to do.

Make sure to warm up before doing these routines to avoid injury and to get the maximum benefit.

Routine 1: Leg and Hip Strengtheners

You need a chair for this routine—sometimes for sitting and sometimes for support. Make sure the chair is sturdy, doesn't wobble, and has a back that you can lean on.

1. **Leg Lifts**

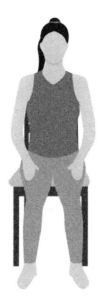 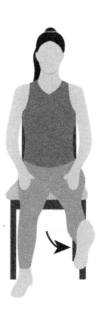

This exercise works your thighs and stretches your hamstrings at the same time, making you stronger and more flexible. Initiate movement from your core command center.

> ➤ Sit in alignment at the front of your chair with your hands resting on your thighs and your feet flat on the floor. Brace your core.

➤ Lift your right leg straight out in front of you, toes pointing toward the ceiling.

➤ Return your foot to the floor. Use the same control you used for your arms in Chapter 4.

➤ Repeat for a total of 10 on your right leg

➤ Take a couple of recovery breaths and check your posture.

➤ Complete 10 lifts on your left leg.

Do a little more: with your leg lifted, give a little extra flex with your foot before you lower it back to the floor.

If your leg doesn't want to come up so that it is parallel to the floor, that is okay. Lift it up as straight as you can, add the little flex, and lower it. As you continue to do the exercise over time, both your strength and flexibility will increase, and you will be able to lift it higher.

2. **Squats**

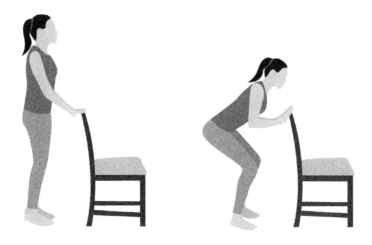

As you squat and work your glutes and thighs, keep part of your focus on the alignment of your skull—make sure it stays in bobble-head position and does not rock back or fall forward.

> ➢ Stand in alignment behind your chair with your feet slightly wider than hip distance and your hands resting lightly on the chair's back for balance. Inhale.

> ➢ As you exhale, push your belly button to your spine and bend your knees as though you were going to sit down. Hinge forward at the hip joints.

> ➢ Sink down as far as you can, using the whole exhale to get there, feeling your weight in your heels, not your back.

> ➢ As you inhale, push against the floor with the bottoms of your feet and rise back up to starting position.

> ➢ Repeat for a total of 10, resting after 5.

You will probably grip the chair's back harder once you are in the squat. That is okay; it helps with balance. However, don't use your hands to help you rise back up—use the muscles of your legs. Thinking of pushing against the floor with your feet helps with this.

Check your position—once you are in the squat, look down. Your knees should be directly above the tops of your feet. If your knees are any farther, or if your heels leave the floor and you come up on your toes, you have gone down too far. Only go as far as you can go with your feet flat on the floor.

3. Back Leg Extensions

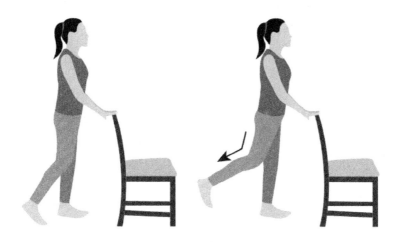

Working your glutes (gluteus maximus) not only gives you a nice, toned bottom, it also helps them do their primary job: supporting the lower spine and stabilizing the hip joints. Weak glutes can lead to problems like lower back and hip pain, difficulty maintaining good posture (so also neck and shoulder pain), and trouble with balance. Don't neglect the glutes!

> ➢ Stand in alignment behind your chair with your feet hip distance apart and your hands on the chair's back for balance.

> ➢ Extend your right leg back and put your toe on the floor. Make sure you have your balance in this position. Adjust as needed to ensure balance before going on.

> ➤ Breathing easily (but still bracing your core), lift your toe off the floor as high as it will go, bring your heel toward the ceiling, and then return your toe to the floor.

> ➤ Repeat for a total of 10; then, do the left leg.

When you lift your leg backward, your knee will be slightly bent. Keep it in the position it was in when your toe was on the floor. Don't bend your knee when you lift your toe to make your foot go higher. How high your foot goes is not important. It may feel like a tiny move, but what is important is that you feel that little burn in your bottom.

Do not lock the knee in your standing leg. Keep that knee soft and slightly bent.

4. **Leg Curl**

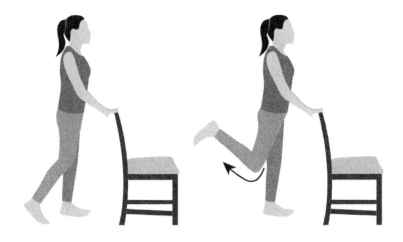

Find your balance for this exercise by shifting your weight so that you can stand on one leg.

> ➢ Stand in alignment behind your chair with your feet hip distance apart and your hands resting on the back of the chair for balance.

> ➢ Shift your weight to your left leg as you prepare to work your right leg. Brace your core.

> ➢ Leave your right thigh hanging and lift your right foot toward your bottom like you're kissing a sailor.

> ➢ Lower your foot to rest on your toes for a second or two and then lift it again.

> ➢ Repeat for a total of 10 curls on each side, resting after five if needed.

Breathe easily with your core braced.

When your leg is as far up as it's going to go, give it an extra little squeeze before you lower again for faster results.

5. **Heel Raises**

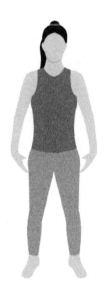 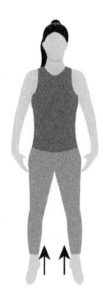

The final exercise of this routine will work your ankle flexors and calf muscles. When you're done, you will have worked every muscle in your legs!

> ➤ Stand in alignment next to your chair. Put one hand on the chair's back for extra balance if you need it. If not, let your arms hang at your sides.

> ➤ Being mindful to keep your posture with your shoulders relaxed down, brace your core and raise up on your toes like you want to see over a tall fence.

> ➤ Return to the floor. Repeat for a total of 10.

> ➤ On the tenth Heel Raise, stay up on your toes for a count of 5 before you come back down and release your core.

Keep the movement slow and steady for the first ten to really work your balance. Then, if you want to give those calves a workout, do ten more twice as fast! The slower you go, the more you work your balance. The faster you go, the more you work your calves!

6. **March in Place**

March for a count of 20 (10 knee lifts on each side) to end this routine with some gentle movement and to get all of those leg muscles working together instead of in isolation. Remember to swing your arms, too!

Routine 2: Legs, Hips, and Balance

This routine is a bit more intense and adds balance work at the end. Have your chair and a bottle of water handy. You work your core and your glutes as well as your leg muscles! Take your time. If you can't do as many repetitions as recommended, remember that's okay. You can build up to it over time. It is better to do fewer repetitions slowly and correctly to get deep into the muscles than to do more repetitions quickly and only have a superficial effect.

1. Side Leg Swings

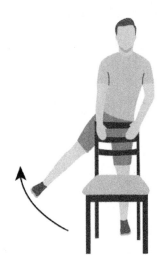 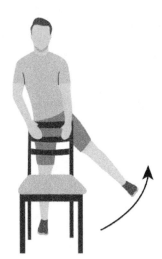

This is great for flexibility in your hips.

➤ Stand in alignment behind your chair with your hands resting on the chair's back for balance.

➤ Shift your weight to your left leg in preparation to lift your right leg. Brace your core.

➤ Lift your right leg out to the side as far as it will go and then bring your foot back to the floor. Control that movement!

➤ Repeat for a total of 12 on each leg.

Keep your foot lightly flexed (in the same position as it was when standing on the floor) as your raise your leg.

Make the motion one slow, sustained motion out and back. There is no need to hold your leg out there. If you want to use your breath for this, complete the pendulum motion during one exhale.

Even though you are balancing on one leg, remember to stay aligned with your ears pointing toward the ceiling and your shoulders relaxed down.

If twelve in a row is too many, try doing six on each leg and then repeat for a total of twelve.

2. **Toe and Heel Raises**

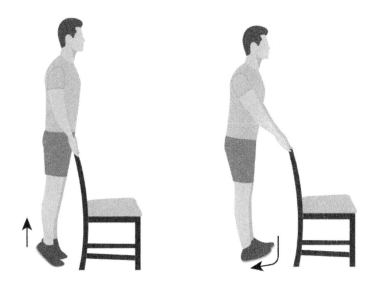

This is like the Heel Raises exercise in the previous routine but adds a toe raise for flexion, hamstrings, and balance.

➤ Stand in alignment behind your chair with your hands resting lightly on the chair's back for balance.

➤ Being mindful to keep your posture and your shoulders relaxed down, breathe easily and raise up on your toes.

➤ Return to the floor and lift your toes off the floor so that you balance on your heels.

➤ Return to standing.

➤ Repeat for a total of 12.

You will naturally bend a little at the waist when you balance back on your heels. That is fine, but try to bend at the waist as little as possible. This will give you a better stretch at the back of your legs.

3. **Reverse Lunges**

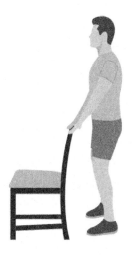 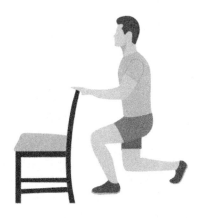

You are about to work all of it! Take your time and use your breath—it will give you more strength and support.

> ➢ Stand in alignment behind your chair with your hands resting on the chair's back for balance. Inhale.

> ➢ As you exhale, engage your core and take a giant step back with your right foot. Bend your left knee to accommodate this movement.

> ➢ As you complete your exhale, press your right heel toward the floor. If it touches the floor, great! If not, that's okay, you'll still feel a great stretch in your calf.

> ➢ Inhale and feel that stretch.

> ➢ As you exhale, brace your core, bend your right knee, and bring it toward the floor. Your left knee will also bend to accommodate this movement.

> ➢ As you inhale, return to your previous position, pressing your heel toward the floor.

> ➢ As you exhale, return to standing.

> ➢ Inhale and get ready to lunge on the other leg.

> ➢ Repeat for a total of 10, five lunges on each leg.

You may not feel that your knee is going very far when you bend it to bring it toward the floor. If you look down, however, you will probably find that your knee is parallel to the floor—which is exactly where you want it to be! Don't try to bring your knee all the way to the floor.

4. **Sit and Stand**

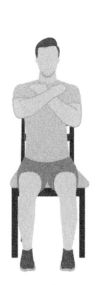
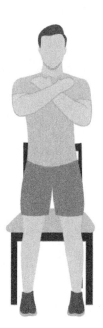

You sit and stand every day, but this exercise gives you practice in doing so properly without creating strain in your back or your neck, which is something people do habitually every day, unknowingly adding to their quota of aches and pains. Keeping proper alignment is key, so let's practice that first.

> ➤ Sit comfortably in your chair and in alignment. Make sure your head is adjusted by rocking it gently forward and back, bringing it to that place of no stress/no stretch, and pulling up on your ears to be doubly sure.

> ➤ Make sure your shoulders are relaxed down. Take a moment or two to close your eyes and visualize your

earlobes and shoulders moving away from each other to get them as relaxed as possible.

➢ Cross your arms over your chest like Dracula to remind your shoulders not to get involved with the upcoming movement.

➢ Hinge at the hips and lean forward and back a few times, making sure that your skull and spine and neck and shoulders stay where they are. The only muscle you should feel engaged is your lower abs.

➢ When you are sure that you can hinge forward and back without any change to your alignment or by involving any muscles but your lower abs, you are ready to stand. Inhale.

➢ As you exhale, hinge forward in the same way, press your feet into the floor, engage your leg muscles, and stand. As you stand, straighten up by hinging back (exactly the same way you did when you were seated).

➢ Good job! Inhale and prepare to sit.

➢ Before you sit, make sure that the chair is right there, close to the backs of your knees. Many people reach with their bottoms to make sure a chair is there before sitting. See that the chair is there so that you do not do that.

➢ Reverse the process of standing: hinge forward and bend your knees slightly; sit easily in the chair you know is there and hinge back to your upright posture.

➢ Repeat for a total of 10.

This should feel like the easiest sitting and standing you have ever done. People engage so many unnecessary muscles when they sit or stand, creating tension that becomes chronic pain. Just think about how many times a day you sit or stand! That's a lot of built-up tension.

Reaching back with your bottom to be sure of the chair throws you out of alignment and adversely affects your lower back. If you do this, stop this habit immediately! Your lower back will thank you.

You should be able to stand by engaging ONLY your core and lower body muscles. Everything above the waist is just along for the ride. However, many people stretch forward with their heads when they go to stand up, creating tension. Your head cannot help you stand up! Working on your alignment at the same time that you work on your leg and core strength will alleviate chronic pain better than any medication.

5. **Toe Taps**

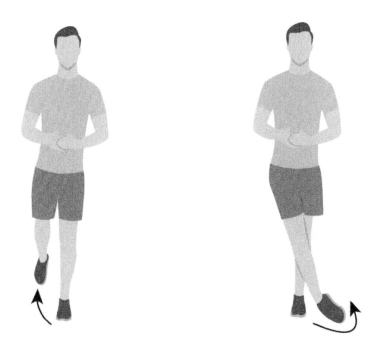

Now that you are standing again, let's work on balance. You can have a chair next to you for support, but try to do this exercise without holding on. If you can't, that's fine—as always; you can work up to it!

> ➢ Stand in alignment with your weight evenly distributed next to your chair's back in case you need to reach out for support.

> ➢ Shift your balance to your left leg.

> ➢ Swing your right foot forward and tap the floor in front of you.

➢ Bring your right foot back and tap the floor next to your left foot.

➢ Swing your right foot back and tap the floor behind you.

➢ Bring your right foot back and tap the floor next to your left foot.

➢ Swing your right foot out to the side and tap the floor to your right.

➢ Bring your right foot back and tap the floor next to your left foot.

➢ Cross your right foot over your left foot and tap the floor over there.

➢ Bring your right foot back to starting position, standing on the floor with your weight evenly distributed.

➢ That's one set. Continue working with your right foot for a total of 8 sets.

➢ Repeat on the left side.

You don't have to come to a standstill between sets; just tap and keep going.

Keep your upper body alignment as your legs are working.

When you can do 8 sets, increase to 10, then 12, and so on up to 20.

6. Balance with Feet Close Together

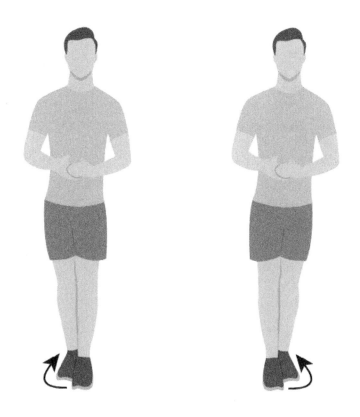

This is harder than it looks and great balance practice! Stand next to your chair in case you need to reach out for support, but try to get to the end without reaching out to steady yourself. Use a timer, or you can count Mississippi's.

➢ Stand in alignment next to your chair.

➢ Place your feet together so that they are touching, with your right foot a little behind your left: the heel of your left foot should be snuggled into the arch of your right foot.

➤ Stand in this position for 60 seconds, and maintain your posture.

➤ Reverse your feet and repeat.

➤ Reverse and repeat with your eyes closed.

It is helpful to find a spot on the wall to stare at if you start to feel wobbly. You always have the option to reach out and steady yourself on the chair, but try staring down your wall first.

Do not lock your knees—keep them soft and unlocked.

Challenge: when you can do this easily, move your front foot forward so that your heel is next to your toe. Finally, place your feet so that one is directly in front of the other, heel touching toe.

Whew! Are those legs feeling stronger? You bet! Balance takes an immense amount of muscle coordination all over your body. Good job working on yours.

CHAPTER 6

The Workout—Back and Chest

G enerally, the back and chest work together, so even though each of these routines actively target muscle groups in front and back, it is inevitable that both back and chest will be working at the same time—a twofer!

Back muscles are arguably the most important muscles in the body. They support the spine and allow the torso to move, bend, and twist. They connect everything from the neck down to the bottom. There are seven muscle groups in the back starting with the trapezius at the top, which connects the neck to the mid-spine. The erector spinae is the lowest muscle in the back. It is one of the major core muscles and runs parallel to the spine from the neck all the way down to connect to the sacrum in the pelvis. Other back muscles you may have heard of include the rhomboids and deltoids.

Strengthening these muscles will help improve posture, ease lower back pain, and reduce stiffness. Let's get started!

Routine 1: Gentle Back Workout

1. **Elbows In**

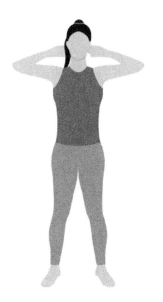 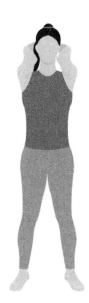

➤ Sit or stand in alignment and place your fingertips lightly behind your head, opening your elbows out to the side.

➤ As you exhale, press your belly button to your spine and slowly bring your elbows toward the center (they may not touch, but you can try).

➢ At the end of your exhale, give an extra little squeeze and see how close you can get (they might even touch!).

➢ As you inhale, open them back out again.

➢ Repeat for a total of 8.

➢ Recover with a couple of Shoulder Rolls.

Don't grip your neck or skull with your hands. Placing your fingers lightly back there just gives you an anchor point for your hands and gets your arms up at the proper angle.

Absolutely stay mindful of your head's position on your neck—in perfect alignment.

2. **Spine Relaxer**

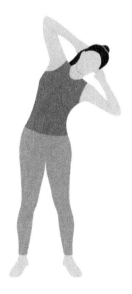 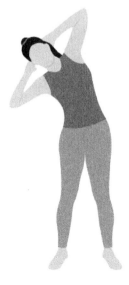

You will remember this exercise from the Seated Core Exercises. It's a great way to follow up the hard work you just did with your elbows.

➢ Sit or stand in alignment with your fingertips lightly behind your head and your elbows open out to the side as in Elbows In. Inhale. Brace your core.

➢ Slowly and gently, lean to the right and think about pointing your left elbow toward the ceiling.

➢ Come back up to standing, taking it slow.

➢ Repeat to the left and so on for a count of 10 (five bends to each side).

If you experience a hitch in your side as you stand back up, you have leaned over too far. As you continue, don't lean over quite as far.

3. Shoulder Rolls

Complete 10 shoulder rolls, breathing easily, and being mindful of your alignment. It feels good to bring those shoulders back and down, doesn't it?

4. Reach for the Sky

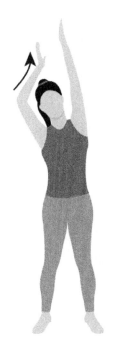 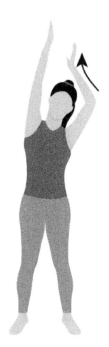

- ➢ Sit or stand in alignment and bring your arms up over your head, palms facing each other. Inhale.

- ➢ Engage your core and stretch your right hand up toward the ceiling for a full exhale.

- ➢ Bring your arms back parallel as you inhale.

- ➢ Repeat on your left, stretching up for the full exhale.

- ➢ Count 20 for ten full stretches up on each side.

- ➢ Finish by breathing easily, counting 10, and reaching up, side to side without pauses so that the movement is continuous.

➤ Lower your arms and shake them out.

It is nice to sigh out your breath while exhaling during this exercise—it makes it feel very relaxing even though you are working your muscles.

5. Low Shoulder Blade Squeeze

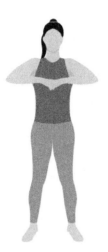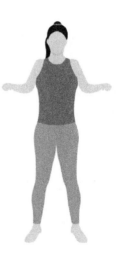

This is a modified version of the Shoulder Blade Squeeze presented in the warmup Stretch Routine. This time, you will not raise your shoulders first but pay close attention to keeping your shoulders relaxed down for the entire movement. They may want to raise up, but you can keep them lowered if you pay attention.

➤ Sit or stand in alignment with your fists pressed together in front of your chest.

- ➢ Imagine that there is a ball hovering between the bottoms of your shoulder blades.

- ➢ As you exhale, gently move your elbows toward your back and try to trap the ball.

- ➢ Bring your fists back together as you inhale.

- ➢ Repeat for a total of 8.

6. **Seated or Standing Cat/Cow**

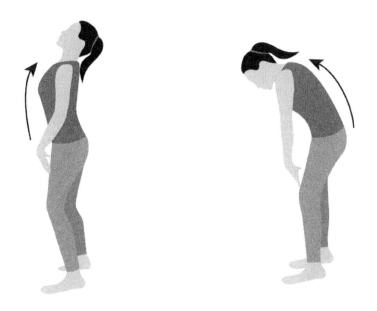

Doing both positions in Cat/Cow while upright is safe because you don't have gravity and the full weight of your belly pulling down on your lower spine. This is a modification of the yoga classic that is great for seniors and people with lower back problems.

> Sit or stand in alignment, hands resting on your thighs.

> As you inhale, gently raise your chin to look at the ceiling and arch your back.

> As you exhale, round over to the front, bringing your chin toward your chest, pressing your belly button toward your spine, and arching your back like that angry Halloween cat.

> Release your abs as you inhale and return to starting position.

> Take a recovery breath.

> Repeat for a total of 5.

7. **Gentle Back Bend**

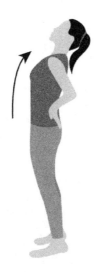 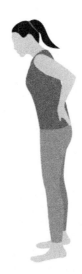

➤ Sit or stand in alignment with your hands at the small of your back for support—palms at the bottom of your ribs and fingers pointing down on your glutes. Inhale.

➤ As you exhale, brace your core.

➤ Raise your chin to look at the ceiling and gently arch your back.

➤ As you inhale, come back to standing (or sitting) in alignment.

➤ Repeat for a total of 5.

It is important to engage your core before beginning the back bend. You want your abs to support this movement, which is designed to make your spine supple. If you don't feel your abs working as you bend back, you have not engaged them enough.

8. Giant Arcs to Heaven

Finish this routine with three or four Giant Arcs to Heaven (like we did in Chapter 2).

➤ Sit or stand in alignment with your arms hanging at your sides.

➤ Inhale and raise your arms out to the side and up over your head.

➤ Exhale and lower your arms back to your sides in the same arc.

➤ Inhale: up. Exhale: down. And you're done!

Routine 2: Chest Workout

When I talk about working the chest muscles, I am talking about the pectoral muscles, which are the most important muscles for the stability and healthy operation of the shoulder joints. They extend across the mass of the chest all the way up to the collarbones and out to connect to the upper arm bones. Although they are not part of the core, they are one of the largest muscles in the upper body. Therefore, they contribute to good posture as well as help with deep breathing because they are attached to the ribs. The ribs have to expand with the breath, and bones cannot do that without healthy muscles to help. We use our pectoral muscles every day when we do things like lift a cup of coffee, squeeze a bottle of shampoo, or push a closet door closed.

You can do these exercises seated or standing, but I recommend that people with lower back problems sit for Presses.

1. **Presses**

   ➤ Sit in alignment at the front of your chair with your feet flat on the floor.

   ➤ Keeping your alignment, hinge forward and lean your left forearm on your left thigh.

   ➤ Extend your right arm so that your fingers are pointing toward the floor to the right of your left foot. This is starting position. Brace your core.

- ➢ Flex your wrist and pull your right elbow back and up toward the ceiling, allowing your chest to rotate with the movement, opening your chest.

- ➢ Lower your right hand back to starting position by pressing the air with your flat palm.

- ➢ Repeat for a total of 15; then, do 15 on the other side.

You may hear some popping in your elbow as you get started. As long as it is a pop with no pain, that's fine. It is just your joint adjusting to this new movement.

2. Genie is a Highchair

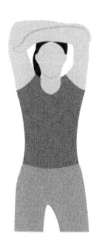 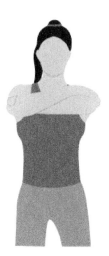

What does that mean? Let's get started and find out!

- ➢ Sit or stand in alignment.

- ➢ Raise your arms in front of you like a genie about to grant a wish.

➢ Turn your bottom hand over so that you can hold onto your forearms with both hands. This is your highchair table. Brace your core.

➢ Breathing easily, raise your highchair table over your head.

➢ Bring it back down in front of your chest.

➢ Repeat for a total of 15 raises.

Although you will be tempted to, do NOT thrust your head forward to get it through your arms. Your head should stay relaxed and in bobble-head position. Do all of the work with your arms and chest muscles.

If you can't get your arms all the way over your head at first, go as far as you can. Your range of motion will increase over time as you continue to do the exercise.

3. **Elbow Press**

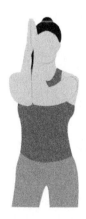
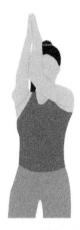

- ➢ Sit or stand in alignment and bring your palms together.

- ➢ Raise your palms until your elbows meet. This is starting position. Brace your core.

- ➢ Breathing easily, separate your elbows and then press them back together.

- ➢ Separate them again and raise your palms so that the bottoms of your hands are at the level of your forehead.

- ➢ Squeeze your elbows together at this higher altitude, separate them, and then lower to the first position.

- ➢ This is one set: one low squeeze followed by one high squeeze.

- ➢ Repeat for a total of 15 sets.

If raising your hands to forehead height is too difficult, do the exercise in the lower position at first. Do 30 squeezes if you stay at the lower level (or build up to 30) and then add the second level.

4. Elbow Kisses

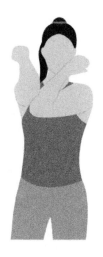 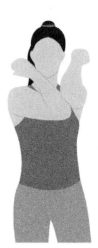

> ➤ Sit or stand in alignment and bring your fists together in front of your chest.

> ➤ Rotate your arms so that your elbows meet.

> ➤ Raise your right elbow about an inch and tap (kiss) your left forearm just above the joint.

> ➤ Switch positions with your left elbow about an inch higher than your right and tap your right forearm just above the joint.

> ➤ Alternate taps for a count of 60 (thirty taps with each elbow), breathing easily with your core braced as you work.

While your elbows are busy trading kisses, remind your shoulders to lower and your head to stay aligned.

5. **Pec Squeeze**

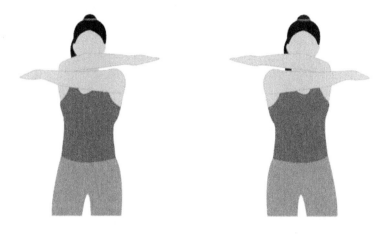

➤ Sit or stand in alignment and bring your flat palms in front of your chest so that your middle fingers meet and your palms face the floor.

➤ Raise your right hand slightly higher than your left.

➤ Move both arms past each other so that your arms cross in front of your chest.

➤ Move them over until your right elbow joint hovers just above your left elbow joint.

➤ Release the squeeze slightly, and then squeeze them again.

➤ Separate your arms so that you can repeat the movement, this time with your left hand hovering over your right.

> ➤ With your core braced, breathe easily and alternate arms for a count of 24, twelve with each arm on top.

The squeezes do not have to last long; they should feel like pulses. If 24 is too many, start with sixteen and work your way up.

6. Chest Opener

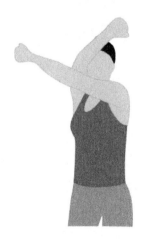 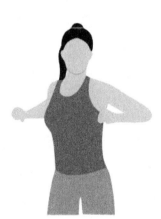

After all that squeezing, let's do the opposite and open up the chest!

> ➤ Sit or stand in alignment so that your wrists cross just in front of your chest, palms open, left closest to your chest. This is starting position.

> ➤ Raise both arms, crossed in an X, until your elbows meet—your crossed elbows should be right in front of your face.

- ➤ Imagine that you are grabbing something you really want and close your fists.

- ➤ Pull back and down so that your elbows go behind your back, and your chest is stretched fully open (you will feel your shoulder blades come together).

- ➤ When you finish pulling back, your fists should be even with your mid-chest, and your shoulders should be dropped.

- ➤ Reach all the way up again to catch another treat, this time with your left arm on the outside and your right arm closest to your chest.

- ➤ Pull your elbows back and down again as before.

- ➤ With your core braced, breathe easily and alternate arms for a count of 24, twelve with each arm on the outside.

Once you get started, this should be a continuous motion up and back. As always, if 24 is too many, start with twelve or sixteen and work your way up.

7. Wall Pushouts

There is no better exercise for the chest muscles than push ups. If you haven't been doing push ups regularly since junior high school, however, they are difficult to impossible to perform. Thank goodness for walls. You can get the same benefit for your chest and arms without straining your back, and you can do more!

➢ Stand in alignment with your feet hip-width apart about a foot from the wall (facing the wall).

➢ Place your palms on the wall at shoulder height and a little more than shoulder width apart. Brace your core.

➢ Keeping your alignment and your body straight as a board, bend your elbows and bring your nose toward the wall until it is almost touching.

➢ Push against the wall with your hands to complete one pushout.

➢ Repeat for a total of 12.

Don't extend your neck to get your nose to the wall faster; keep your head aligned always.

Play around with your hand position to find the most comfortable and beneficial placement for you.

Challenge yourself by taking an extra, normal-sized step back away from the wall and doing 12 more pushouts.

It is so great to be able to get the benefit of push ups without the strain of having to plank. If, however, you decide to do regular pushups instead of wall pushouts, remember that engaging your core is essential to protecting your lower back.

As I am sure you noticed, these exercises worked not only the chest muscles but the arm and back muscles, as well. Wall Pushouts even work the flexion in your ankles! Isn't it nice to know that even when you target a certain muscle group, multiple muscles all over your body benefit?

CHAPTER 7

The Workout—Cardiovascular

C ardiovascular exercise means aerobics. Aerobics calls to mind images of Jane Fonda jumping around in her little striped shirt or of Richard Simmons sweating to the oldies in his little striped shorts. Yes, aerobics have been popular ever since science pinpointed the advantages of regular cardiovascular exercise. According to doctors at the Mayo Clinic (Mayo Clinic Staff, 2020), who recommend at least 2 ½ hours of cardio per week, those advantages include:

➢ Losing weight and keeping it off

➢ Increasing stamina and reducing fatigue from everyday activities

➢ Improving the immune system to help ward off colds and flu

➢ Lowering blood pressure and controlling blood sugar

➢ Reducing the pain of arthritis

➢ Managing coronary artery disease

➢ Strengthening your heart muscle

➢ Boosting good cholesterol and lowering bad cholesterol

➢ Promoting relaxation and improving sleep

➢ Easing depression and anxiety; improving your mood

➢ Maintaining mobility and independence

➢ Lowering the risk of falls and other injuries

➢ Protecting memory and preventing dementia

➢ Extending life expectancy

That's a lot of benefit from 2 ½ hours of cardio per week!

What counts as aerobic exercise? The word aerobic comes from two Greek roots: "aer" meaning air and "bios" meaning life. Any exercise that increases your heart rate from your normal resting heart rate and causes you to breathe more deeply is aerobic exercise. Aerobic exercises are also often defined as "with air" because you increase your oxygen intake while performing them. Increasing oxygen helps to strengthen muscles!

How will I know when I have increased my heartrate enough? You will feel your heart beating a bit faster than usual, and you will notice that your breathing deepens. However, you should not feel out of breath or feel your heart pounding. If you cannot continue what you are doing and still hold a conversation, you are doing too much too soon and need to slow down.

What happens in my body during aerobic exercise? Breathing faster and more deeply increases the amount of oxygen in the blood. Your faster heart rate decreases the amount of time it takes for your blood to bring oxygen to your muscles. Your capillaries (small blood vessels) open wider to bring more blood to your muscles and whisk away toxins. And finally, your body releases endorphins that make you feel great by reducing pain and increasing feelings of wellbeing (Mayo Clinic Staff, 2020).

What is the difference between low-impact and high-impact aerobics? Impact refers to the burden on bones and joints. Activities like running or jumping cause more pressure and jarring, so they are high-impact. Activities like walking or swimming cause minimal pressure and jarring to bones and joints, so they are low-impact. Low-impact aerobic exercise is recommended for seniors, people recovering from injury, and people unaccustomed to regular, vigorous exercise.

How can I get my two-and-a-half hours of cardio a week? There are two low-impact cardio workouts in this book: Belly Fat Exercises in Chapter 3 and the workout below. You will also find that some of the other workout routines that target specific muscle groups increase your breathing and heart rate, too. They also count as cardio! A nice walk or trip to the pool can also help you add up those cardio minutes.

The key to a great cardio workout is to *never stop moving.* As you transition from one movement to the next, march in between. If you begin to breathe too hard, or your heart begins to beat too fast, *slow down* but stop only if you begin to feel dizzy or nauseous. Now, grab a bottle of water, put on some fun music, and let's get moving!

Cardio Workout

1. **March in Place**

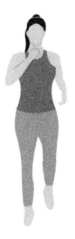 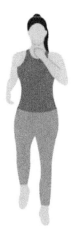

March in place to the beat of your music for a minute, bringing your knees up and pumping your arms to slowly begin to increase your heart rate.

You do not have to bring your knees up to 90°; about half that is just right.

Maintain your aligned posture with your core engaged and your shoulders relaxed down!

Breathe in through your nose and out through your mouth.

2. **Add 4 Giant Arcs to Heaven** (see Chapter 2)

➤ Inhale and raise your arms up over your head.

➤ Exhale and lower your arms back down.

➤ Repeat for a total of 4. Don't stop marching!

March in Place for 30 seconds. Don't forget to pump your arms!

3. **Heel Taps Forward**

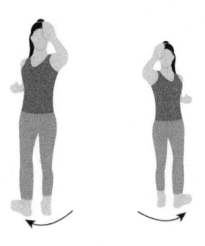

➢ Using the beat of your music, transition from marching to extending your heels forward and tapping the floor.

➢ When you are moving easily tapping your heels, add your arms by pressing your palms directly out in front of you.

➢ Press with your right palm when you tap with your left foot and vice versa.

➢ Continue for a count of 30 (fifteen presses forward with each hand).

March in Place for 30 seconds.

4. **Toe Taps Side**

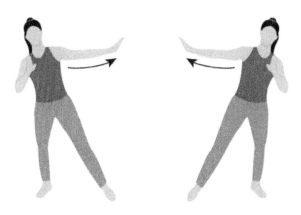

➢ Transition from marching to extending your toes to tap out to your sides.

➢ When you are moving easily, add your arms by pressing your palm out to the side in the same direction that you are tapping.

➢ Continue for a count of 30 (fifteen presses with each hand).

March in Place for <u>20</u> seconds.

5. **Toe Taps Back**

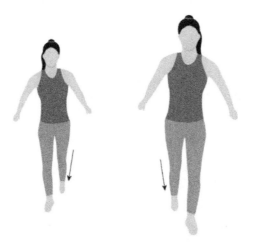

➢ Transition from marching to extending your feet behind you to tap the floor.

➢ When you are moving easily, add your arms by closing your fists and swinging your arms back with each toe tap. Do not keep your arms straight. Bend your elbows and initiate the arm movement from there.

➢ Continue for a count of 30 arm swings back.

March in Place for 20 seconds.

6. **March Up and Back**

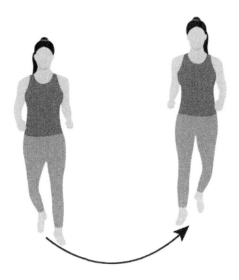

➢ Transition from marching in place to marching forward four steps and then marching backward four steps.

➢ Continue for a total of 8 trips front and back.

➢ A good way to count this is (forward) **1**-2-3-4, (back) 5-6-7-8; (forward) **2**-2-3-4, (back) 5-6-7-**8**; (forward) **3**-2-3-4, and so on.

March in Place for 20 seconds.

7. Step and Tap Side to Side

➤ Transition from marching by stepping right.

➤ Close the space you made by bringing your left foot over and tapping the floor next to your right foot.

➤ Step left onto your left foot, close the space and tap with your right foot. Continue to the beat of your music.

➤ When you are comfortable with this movement, add your arms by reaching out with your fists and pulling your elbows back to your sides with each tap.

➤ Continue for a total of 30, counting one for each tap.

March in Place for <u>10</u> seconds.

8. Arm Extensions Up and Down

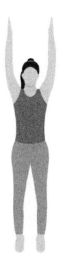
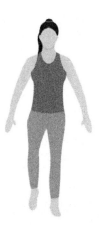

- Keep marching and add your arms.

- Reach up with your arms like a toddler getting his shirt removed.

- Lower your arms like you're dropping something heavy on the ground.

- Each up and down movement of your arms should take four march steps.

- Continue for a total of 15, counting each time you reach overhead.

March in Place for 20 seconds.

9. **Kick Out**

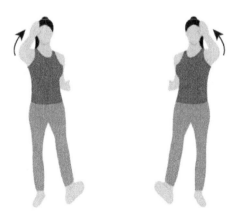

- This is like Heel Taps but you do not touch your heel to the floor.

➤ Add your arms in the same way as Heel Taps by pressing your palm forward at chest height as you kick out using opposites: kick with your left foot and press with your right hand.

➤ Continue for a total of 30 kicks (fifteen with each foot)

March in Place for 10 seconds.

10. **Tap** and **Push**

➤ Transition from marching to extending your toes to tap to your sides.

➤ When you are moving easily, add your arms by pressing your palm across your body: tap with your right foot and press your right palm across your body to the left.

➤ Turn your torso slightly to accommodate the movement of your arms.

➤ Continue for a count of 30 (fifteen presses with each hand).

March in Place for 10 seconds.

11. **Leg Curls**

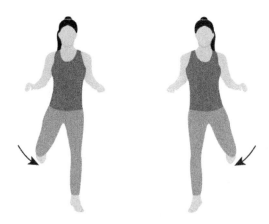

> ➤ Transition from marching to shifting your weight so that you can lift a foot off the floor. You will need a wide stance for this.

> ➤ Bend your knee and kick your foot up toward your bottom as in Leg Curls (Chapter 5 —"kiss the sailor").

> ➤ When you are curling in time to your music, add your arms by reaching out for some invisible taffy in front of you and pulling your elbows back behind you. One pull back for each Leg Curl.

> ➤ Continue for a total of 30 taffy pulls (fifteen on each leg).

March in Place for 10 seconds.

12. Double Side Step

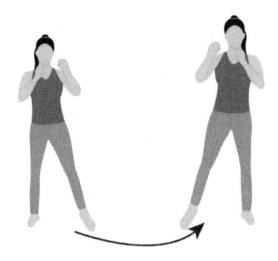

➢ Transition from marching to taking two steps to the side.

➢ Step right on your right foot.

➢ Close that space with your left foot.

➢ Step right again on your right foot.

➢ With your left foot, close that space, tap, and step left.

➢ Close that space with your right foot.

➢ Step left again on your left foot.

➢ With your right foot, close that space, tap, and step right.

- Swing your arms forward and back, elbows bent, with the movement.

- Continue for a total of 20, counting each time you change direction (1=double step right, 2=double step left, etc.).

March in Place for <u>20</u> seconds.

13. **Grapevine**

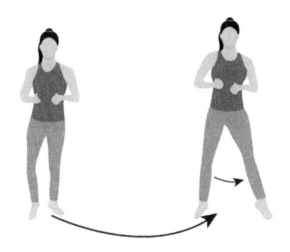

- Transition from marching to taking two steps to the side.

- Step right on your right foot.

- Step right with your left foot, crossing your left foot behind your right foot.

- Step right again with your right foot.

- Close the space with your left foot and tap.

- Step left on your left foot.

- Step left with your right foot, crossing your right behind your left foot.

- Step left again with your left foot.

- Close the space with your right foot and tap.

- Swing your arms forward and back, elbows bent, as in Double Side Step.

- Continue for a total of 20, counting each time you change direction.

March in Place for 20 seconds.

14. V Step

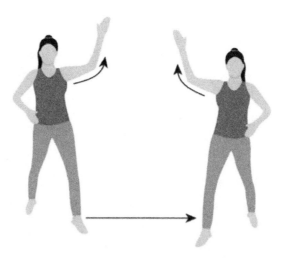

➢ Transition from marching by taking a big step forward and to the right with your right foot.

➢ Bring your left foot up to the level of your right foot and make your stance very wide (this is the top of the V).

➢ Step back and slightly left with your right foot.

➢ Bring your left foot to the side of your right foot. You are now standing at the bottom of your V.

➢ Continue stepping up wide and stepping back with feet together until you are comfortable with the foot movement.

➢ Add your arms: raise your right hand over your head as you step forward on your right foot.

➢ Raise your left hand as you step forward on your left foot.

➢ Lower your right hand to your waist, elbow bent as you step back on your right foot.

➢ Lower your left hand in the same manner as you step back on your left foot.

➢ Continue for a total of 10 Vs starting with the right foot.

➢ Repeat for 10 more starting with the left foot.

March in Place for 20 seconds.

15. **Mambo**

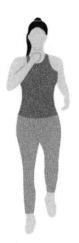 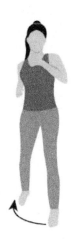

> Transition from marching by moving one leg front to back.

> Step forward on your right foot (stepping on your toe with your heel raised works best).

> Return your weight to your left foot.

> Step backward on your right toe.

> Return your weight to your left foot.

> Repeat by bringing your right foot all the way forward.

> Basically, your left foot stays in place as your right foot moves first in front of you and then behind you.

> Continue to pump your arms as when you march.

- ➢ Mambo for a total of fifteen on your right foot, counting each time your foot comes forward.

- ➢ Repeat on the left.

March in Place for <u>30</u> seconds.

- ➢ Inhale deeply and exhale fully as you begin to slow your march.

- ➢ Stop after 30 seconds.

- ➢ Do 3 Arcs to Heaven with big inhales and exhales to stretch it out and finish.

Great job! This routine will take anywhere from fifteen to twenty-five minutes depending on the tempo of your music. I suggest starting with fun music at a slower tempo until you get the hang of each step and the flow of the routine. Then, transition to music with a faster tempo for a more intense workout.

Remember to monitor your heart rate and breathing. Slow down and just march if you are doing too much. Give your body a chance to recover, and then continue with the routine at a slower pace.

Chapter 8

The Workout—Joints and Joint Pain

─────────────────────────

J oint pain is another condition many people have to contend with as they age. According to doctors at the Cleveland Clinic, joint pain has several causes (Cleveland Clinic, 2018). These causes include:

- Osteoarthritis; occurs when the cartilage cushion between bones wears away.

- Rheumatoid arthritis; occurs when the joints experience swelling and pain.

- Bursitis; occurs when the joints have been overused.

- Tendinitis; occurs when tendons (the fibrous tissue that connects muscle to bone) become inflamed.

- Injuries due to breaks or sprains.

All of these conditions can cause mild to severe joint pain. If you are experiencing joint pain, exercise is one the best ways to help. This is because exercise strengthens the muscles that protect them. In addition to exercise, the orthopedic staff at the Cleveland Clinic recommend the following (Cleveland Clinic, 2020):

- Stop smoking. Smoking increases inflammation. "Within eight hours of quitting, the carbon monoxide level in your blood returns to normal and the oxygen levels in your blood increase" (Cleveland Clinic, 2020). As I said in the previous chapter, increased oxygen levels help build muscle faster, so if you are a smoker, you are sabotaging the good you are trying to do with exercise.

- Drink more water. Water is the main ingredient your body uses to make cartilage. Cartilage cushions your joints. Without enough water, your body will pull water from your cartilage for other needs, leaving your joints without all of the protection they could have. For this reason, plain water is the best drink for your joints—and another reason to stay away from soda.

- Maintain a healthy weight. The more overweight *or* underweight you are, the more pressure and tension on your joints.

Finally, you need to listen to your body when you exercise. It is normal to experience some muscle soreness after exercise. However, if the soreness you feel is *not* in your muscle but in your joints, see your doctor. It may be that there is a problem with the way you are performing the exercise; on the other hand, it may be a symptom of one of the conditions listed above. Make sure your doctor knows what you are doing so that they can correctly diagnose the root of the problem.

Routine 1: Three Shoulder Exercises

Most of these exercises can be done seated or standing.

1. **Triceps Stretch**

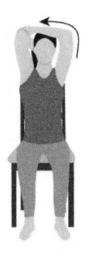 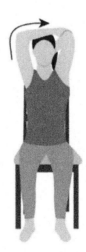

> Sit or stand in alignment.

➢ Slowly raise your left arm over your head and then bend your elbow so that your hand comes down behind your head.

➢ Reach up with your right hand and lightly grip the outside of your left elbow.

➢ Apply pressure with your right hand until you feel the stretch in the outside muscle of your left arm.

➢ Hold the stretch for 30 seconds (about 5 full, deep inhales and exhales).

➢ Focus on relaxing into the stretch as you breathe.

➢ Bring both arms down to your sides and notice the difference in how the two sides feel, paying particular attention to the relaxation in your left shoulder.

➢ Repeat on the other side.

2. **Wings**

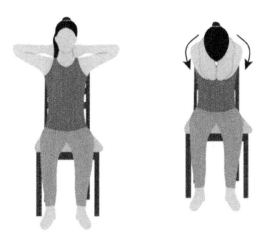

➤ Sit or stand in alignment and place your fingertips lightly at the base of your skull. Inhale.

➤ As you exhale, press your elbows toward the wall behind you.

➤ Hold for another full inhale and exhale. Make sure that you do not press against your head.

➤ Inhale. As you exhale, bring your elbows in front of you and round over forward, dropping your chin toward your chest and your elbow toward your knees. You can leave your fingers lightly touching the base of your skull, but DO NOT pull down on your head.

➤ Feel the stretch going down your neck and into the muscles of your mid-back.

➤ Remain in this position for two complete, relaxing exhales.

➤ Return to sitting in alignment.

➤ Repeat for a total of 3 in each position.

Your head weighs between eight and twelve pounds. That is plenty of weight; just let gravity do its job. You can help it along by relaxing. However, pulling down on your head with your hands is unnecessary and dangerous. Don't do it!

3. Hanging Arm Circles

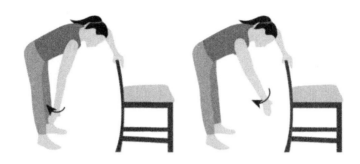

➤ Stand in alignment behind your chair.

➤ Hinge forward at the hips and extend your left arm so that your forearm comes to rest on the back of the chair. Your right arm will hang, relaxed, down toward the floor.

➤ Make sure you are not locking your knees!

➤ Breathing easily, circle your arm clockwise at about the circumference of a salad bowl for a count of 15.

➤ Let your arm come to a hanging standstill.

➤ Circle your arm counterclockwise for a count of 15.

➤ Return to standing by placing both hands on the back of your chair and pushing.

➤ Repeat on the left side.

What a nice, gentle way to end this series!

Routine 2: Hand, Wrist, and Elbow Exercises

Have two tennis balls or other small balls that fit in the palms of your hands ready. If you don't have balls, you can use rolled up socks, beanbags, or anything else that fits the palms of your hands.

1. **Ball Squeezes**

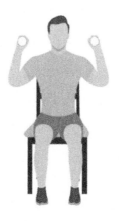 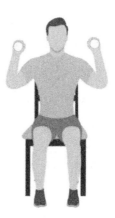

> ➢ Sit in alignment on your chair with a ball in each hand.

> ➢ Raise your hands at chest level with your elbows pointing toward the floor. Inhale.

> ➢ As you exhale, squeeze the balls and count to five. Push your belly button to your spine and make your exhale last the length of the squeeze.

- ➢ Relax and inhale. Take a recovery breath.

- ➢ Repeat for a total of 5 squeezes.

- ➢ Lower your hands and shake out your arms.

Make sure you use all five fingers to squeeze. Maintain your posture—shoulders relaxed back and down and skull in bobble-head position.

2. **Finger Stretches**

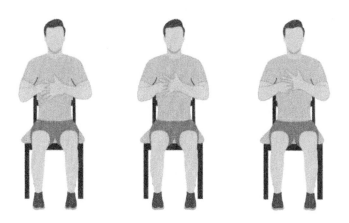

- ➢ Sit in alignment.

- ➢ Raise your left hand so that your fingers are about chest height and relaxed.

- ➢ Raise your right hand so that your index and middle fingers are extended like a closed pair of imaginary scissors.

➢ Place the closed scissors of your right hand between the index and middle fingers of your left hand, down by the knuckle and the middle joint of the fingers. Inhale.

➢ As you exhale, open your scissors to stretch the relaxed index and middle fingers of your left hand.

➢ Count to 5 and make your exhale last the length of the stretch.

➢ Remove your scissors, relax, and take a recovery breath.

➢ Repeat by stretching between your middle finger and ring finger.

➢ Repeat by stretching between your ring finger and your pinky.

➢ Repeat on the other hand.

These exercises are a great opportunity to strengthen your core while you relax and exercise your joints. Take advantage of it by using your breath to engage your core. Of course, you can simply count to five and get the hand work done, but why not simply and easily get two benefits from one exercise?

3. **Open and Close**

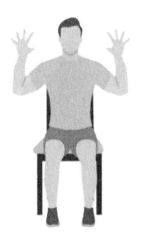 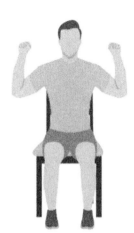

➢ Sit in alignment in your chair and raise your hands beside you with your elbows pointing toward the floor. Inhale.

➢ As you exhale, actively stretch your fingers as wide as they will go.

➢ On a count of five, press your belly button to your spine and stretch those fingers out.

➢ Inhale and lightly close your fists.

➢ As you exhale and push your belly button toward your spine, squeeze your fists as tight as you can, and count to 5.

➢ Inhale and open your hands.

➢ Repeat for a total of 10. If you need to, lower your arms and take a break after 5.

4. **Wrist Flexion**

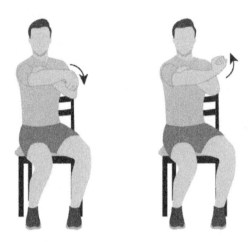

➢ Sit in alignment and extend your left arm out in front of you with your fist closed.

➢ Lightly place your right hand on top of your left arm between the elbow and the shoulder. It is there to remind your shoulder to stay relaxed down.

➢ Breathing easily, slowly and gently flex your wrist so that the knuckles point toward the ceiling. Go as far as you can without pain.

➢ Reverse and flex your wrist so that your knuckles point toward the floor.

➢ Repeat for a total of 8, keeping the movement slow and gentle.

➢ Repeat with the other wrist. Remember to keep your arm straight.

➢ Relax and shake out both arms at your sides to finish.

Modification: if you need help holding your arm out for that long, instead of placing your other hand on top of your upper arm, place it between your elbow and your wrist on the underside to help hold up the arm that is working.

5. **Lateral Wrist Flexion**

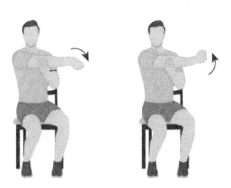

➢ Sit in alignment and extend your left arm out in front of you with your hand open and your thumb pointing toward the ceiling.

➢ Close your fist and bring your right hand underneath to support your left arm at the elbow.

➢ Breathing easily, gently flex your wrist upwards so that your thumb knuckle points back toward your elbow and then forward toward the wall in front of you.

➢ Repeat for a total of 8.

➢ Check to make sure your shoulder remains relaxed down.

➢ Repeat with the other wrist.

➢ Relax and shake it out to finish.

6. **Elbow Stretch**

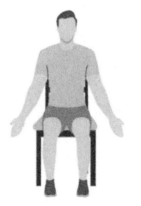 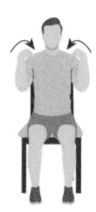

➤ Sit in alignment at the front of your chair and let your arms hang down by your sides. Brace your core.

➤ Bend your elbows and raise your hands to touch your shoulders.

➤ Lower your hands to your sides.

➤ When you reach the bottom, give an extra little press back and feel the muscles on the insides of your elbows stretch.

➤ Lift your hands back to your shoulders and continue for a total of 10. Take a core break after 5 if needed.

7. **Easy Elbow Rotation**

➤ Sit in alignment facing forward.

➤ Raise your arms in front of you with your palms open and facing the floor, but keep your elbows touching the outsides of your ribs.

➤ Breathe easily as you gently rotate your hands so that your palms face up.

➤ Rotate up and down for 10, counting each time your palms turn up.

This exercise resembles Easy Shoulder Rotation in Chapter 4. The difference is that the arms are not extended, so the shoulders don't get involved—only the elbows.

Routine 3: Reduce Knee Pain

The only way to reduce knee pain is to build up the muscles around the joint, so this routine will work the muscles in the legs. Before you do this routine, be sure and warm up using the routine in Chapter 2. As an alternative, you can march in place and pump your arms vigorously for two minutes to get your blood flowing and muscles warmed up. I do not recommend doing this routine with "cold" muscles. Remember that warming up helps prevent injury because it prepares muscles for the work ahead.

8. **Ankle Rolls**

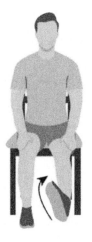 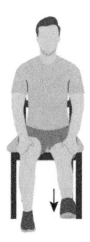

➢ Sit in alignment at the front of your chair with your hands resting on your thighs.

- ➤ Raise your right foot off the floor and gently circle your toes to the right for a count of 10.

- ➤ Reverse and circle your toes to the left for a count of 10.

- ➤ Repeat on the left leg, breathing easily through your nose.

9. **Alternating Leg Lifts**

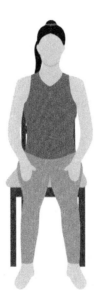 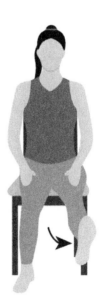

- ➤ Sit in alignment with your hands on your thighs and feet flat on the floor.

- ➤ As you exhale, brace your core and lift your right leg straight out in front of you, toes pointing toward the ceiling.

> As you inhale, release your core and return your foot to the floor.

> Repeat with the left leg.

> Continue for a count of 8, four lifts on each side.

10. Seated March in Place

> Remain seated in your chair and rest your hands either on or in front of your belly. Brace your core.

> Alternate lifting your feet off the floor to march in your chair.

> Remember to maintain your upright and relaxed posture.

> Lift your knees nice and high and remember to pump your arms.

> March for a count of 20, ten lifts on each leg.

You learned the next few exercises in Chapter 5. Instructions are repeated here so that you don't have to turn back. The number of repetitions varies slightly.

11. Squats

> Stand in alignment behind your chair with your feet slightly wider than hip distance and your hands resting on the chair's back for balance. Inhale.

➢ As you exhale, engage your core and bend your knees as though you were going to sit down. Hinge forward at the hip joints.

➢ Sink down as far as you can, using the whole exhale to get there, feeling your weight in your heels, not your back.

➢ As you inhale, push against the floor with the bottoms of your feet and rise back up to starting position.

➢ Repeat for a total of 10, resting after 5 if needed.

12. **Side Leg Swings**

➢ Stand in alignment behind your chair with your hands resting on the chair's back for balance.

➢ Shift your weight to your left leg in preparation to lift your right leg. Brace your core.

➢ Lift your right leg out to the side as far as it will go and then bring your foot back to the floor. Keep your toes facing forward and your foot in the same flexed position as it was when it was on the floor.

➢ Complete 10 lifts on each leg.

13. Sit and Stand

These are abbreviated instructions. If you are doing this routine before you do Routine 2 in Chapter 10, please see the more complete instructions there. Doing this exercise *correctly* will not only strengthen your legs and core, it will also alleviate strain and tension in your neck and upper back.

➢ Sit in alignment.

➢ Cross your arms over your chest like Dracula to remind your shoulders not to get involved.

➢ Hinge at the hips and lean forward and back a few times, making sure there is no change to your alignment. Inhale.

➢ As you exhale, hinge forward, press your feet into the floor, engage your leg muscles, and stand. As you stand, straighten up by hinging back.

➢ Inhale and prepare to sit by making sure the chair is there.

➢ Reverse the process of standing: hinge forward and bend your knees; sit and hinge back to your upright posture.

➢ Repeat for a total of 10.

14. Modified Back Leg Extensions

➤ Stand in alignment behind your chair with your feet hip distance apart and your hands on the chair for balance. Brace your core.

➤ Extend your right leg back, tap your toe on the floor, and return to standing.

➤ Complete 10 extensions on each leg.

15. Downhill Skiing

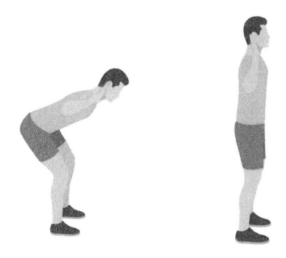

➤ Stand in alignment behind your chair with your feet slightly wider than hip distance apart.

➤ Raise your fists up to the level of your temples. Inhale.

➢ As you exhale, press your belly button to your spine, bend your knees, and hinge forward at the hip joints, sinking back with your bottom to balance.

➢ As you do this, your arms will naturally come down to chest level. Imagine that you are holding ski poles and flying downhill.

➢ As you inhale, hinge back up, and return to standing. Check your alignment before you go again.

➢ Ski down 10 hills.

If you keep your alignment as you hinge forward, you will be looking at the floor in front of your feet. This is the same hinge as Sit and Stand.

Do not bend your knees too deeply. When you are in "racing downhill" position, you should feel a stretch behind your knees. If you don't feel that stretch, you have bent your knees too much. Straighten up slightly by lifting your bottom until you feel the stretch.

Modification: do this exercise with your hands on the back of your chair for balance if you need to. If you do the exercise as instructed, stand behind your chair so that the chair's back is there if you need to reach out for balance.

16. Heel Raises

➢ Stand in alignment next to your chair. Put one or both hands on the chair's back for extra balance if needed. If not, let your arms hang at your sides.

➤ Keeping your posture and with your shoulders relaxed down, breathe easily and raise up on your toes like you want to see over a tall fence.

➤ Return to the floor. Repeat for a total of 10.

➤ On the tenth Heel Raise, stay up on your toes for a count of 5 before you come back down.

17. **Alternating Leg Lifts**

➤ Sit in alignment, hands resting on your thighs, feet flat on the floor. Brace your core.

➤ Lift your right foot straight out in front of you, toes pointing toward the ceiling.

➤ Add that extra tiny flex before returning your right foot to the floor.

➤ Alternate legs for a count of 20, ten lifts for each leg.

18. **Modified Hamstring Stretch**

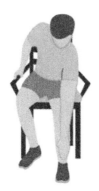 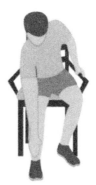

➢ Sit in alignment at the front of your chair with your hands resting on your thighs or arm rest.

➢ Extend your right foot out in front of you and rest your heel on the floor, toes pointing at the ceiling. Inhale.

➢ As you exhale, hinge forward and reach for your toes with your right hand.

➢ Use your other hand for balance.

➢ Use the entire exhale to get as far as you can go; you will feel that friendly ache in the back of your right leg.

➢ When you reach that point, lower the fingertips of your right hand to rest on the top of your lower leg.

➢ Hang out in this position, deepening the stretch, for four more full exhales.

➢ On each exhale, tell yourself to relax and see if your fingertips will move just a tiny bit closer to your foot. Remember—this can only happen if you relax.

➢ When you have completed five full exhales, sit back up as you inhale.

➢ Take a couple of recovery breaths and repeat on your left leg.

Because this is a cool down instead of a warmup, you will hold the position longer and concentrate on relaxing. There should be no pain in the back of your leg—just a deep and healthy stretch in the four muscles that form the hamstrings.

Remember: never push or force when you stretch. Pushing can cause injury. Just breathe and relax!

19. **Gentle Back Bend**

➢ Sit or stand in alignment with your hands at the small of your back for support. Inhale.

➢ As you exhale, gently raise your chin to look at the ceiling and arch your back slightly.

➢ Hold in this position for 5 full exhales and really feel that stretch.

Your breaths do not have to qualify as deep belly breathing here, and you don't have to engage your core. Your aim is to relax and get the benefit of stretching in the opposite direction from the Hamstring Stretch.

If you are standing and feel like you need more support, squeeze your glutes—remember that they are a (minor) core muscle, too!

Routine 4: Seated Hip Workout

If you have a resistance band, it is a great addition to this workout. If you don't, that's okay. You can still do the workout and get significant benefit from it. The first three exercises are a warmup before we get into the strengthening work. Therefore, you may skip the warmup in Chapter 2 before doing this routine.

1. **Seated March in Place**

   ➢ Sit in alignment at the front of your chair, fists on your thighs.

   ➢ Breathe easily as you alternate lifting your feet off the floor to march in your chair.

   ➢ Remember to maintain your upright and relaxed posture.

   ➢ Bring your knees up nice and high and don't forget to pump your arms.

   ➢ March for a count of 40, twenty lifts on each leg.

If a count of forty is not enough to deepen your breathing and get your heartrate up, keep marching until you feel that you have reached an aerobic state. Of course, if you do the warmup in Chapter 2 first, you will already be warmed up and ready to go, so you won't need to add any extra marching.

2. **Glute Stretch**

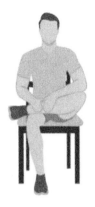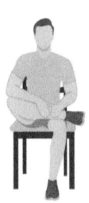

➢ Sit in alignment at the front of your chair and set your right ankle on top of your left knee.

➢ Lightly hold onto your right shin with both hands and rest your right elbow on your right thigh (or just above it). Inhale.

➢ Keeping your alignment, exhale and hinge forward at the hips.

➢ You will feel the stretch in your right hip. Hold here and inhale.

➢ Deepen the stretch by remaining in this position for 5 full exhales.

➢ Each time you exhale, consciously relax and see if you can hinge forward just a fraction more.

➤ Return to sitting upright after your fifth exhale and repeat on your left side.

Keeping your upright posture when you hinge forward is extremely important. If you round your back and bend forward instead of hinging, you will lose the good stretch in your hip. Try it both ways so that you feel the difference. That way, you will know when you are doing it correctly.

If you relax and can't hinge forward any more, that's okay. Just hold the stretch there and keep breathing. You are doing your hip flexors a world of good just by getting into this position!

3. **Inner Thigh Stretch**

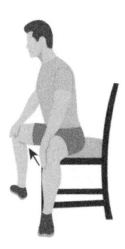

➤ Sit in alignment at the front of your chair and spread your legs so that your knees are pointing out to the sides, making an obtuse angle.

➤ Your feet are flat on the floor, and your toes point the same direction as your knees.

➤ Place your palms on the insides of your legs at the knees.

➤ Feel the stretch in your inner thighs. Use your hands to encourage your legs to stay where they are.

➤ Hold this position for 5 full exhales.

➤ Deepen the stretch when you exhale by pushing your belly button to your spine and pressing your knees outward. They won't actually move, but you will feel that extra little squeeze in your muscles.

➤ Relax when you inhale and squeeze when you exhale.

➤ When you finish your fifth breath, gently release the stretch and slowly bring your knees back to the front of your chair.

Let your feet and legs do whatever they want to recover — let your feet have a little tantrum on the floor in front of your chair!

4. **Hip Flexion**

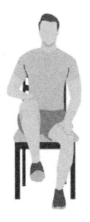 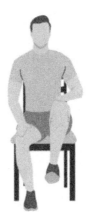

➤ Sit in alignment, feet flat on the floor, hands resting on your knees. Brace your core.

➤ Lift your right knee as high as you can and bring it back to the floor.

➤ Complete 10 lifts on each leg.

5. **Extended Leg Lifts**

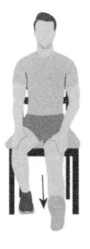 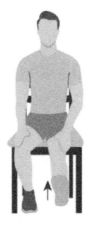

- ➢ Sit in alignment, hands resting on your thighs, right leg extended so that your heel rests on the floor.

- ➢ Brace your core, keep your leg straight, and lift your foot off the floor.

- ➢ Lower your foot to touch the floor and repeat.

- ➢ Compete 10 lifts with each leg.

Bracing your core for exercises four and five will not only help you lift your leg higher, it will also prevent you from leaning back. You don't want to lean back. For maximum benefit and range of motion in your hip, remain seated and upright.

Because this is intended to be a hip exercise rather than a hamstring exercise, stop your upward motion when you feel the muscles in the backs of your legs engage. Lower your leg and continue to work on your hip flexion rather than stretch your hamstrings.

6. **Inner Thigh Squeeze**

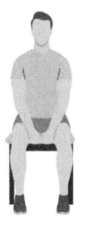
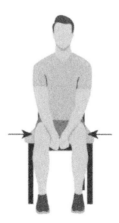

➢ Sit in alignment with your knees slightly apart.

➢ Bring your fists together, knuckles toward the ceiling, and place them between your knees.

➢ Brace your core and squeeze your fists with your knees for a slow count of 5.

➢ Release and take a couple of recovery breaths.

➢ Repeat for a total of 5 squeezes.

Modification: if your hands are too tender to stand being squeezed, you can use a sturdy household item like a medium-sized saucepan instead.

7. **Inner Thigh Press**

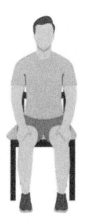 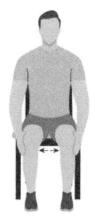

➢ Sit in alignment, knees slightly apart, palms resting out the outsides of your knees. Brace your core.

➢ Push out with your knees and in with your hands for a slow count of five.

➢ Release and take a couple of recovery breaths.

➢ Repeat for a total of 5 presses.

8. **Leg Extensions with Resistance**

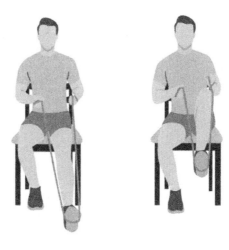

➢ Sit in alignment at the front of your chair and place your resistance band under your right foot. *If you don't have a resistance band, place your hands on the chair's seat behind your hips.*

➢ Lift your right foot off the floor and bring your knee toward your chest, keeping your resistance band tight against your flexed foot. *If you don't have a resistance band, just lift your leg in the same manner.*

➢ Brace your core, press your flexed right foot toward the floor, and straighten it. If you are using a band, pressing your foot out will be harder.

➢ Breathe easily with your core braced for a total of 10 extensions on each leg.

The amount of resistance depends on how much you choke up on your band. Experiment and find a length where you feel like you're getting a good workout but not having to work too hard.

9. **Open and Close with Resistance**

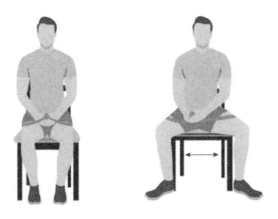

➢ Sit in alignment at the front of your chair, feet flat on the floor.

➢ If you have a resistance band, bring it underneath your thighs and tie it together on top.

➤ Hold onto your resistance band to make sure it doesn't come undone. *If you don't have a band, rest your hands on your thighs.*

➤ Brace your core, lift your feet off the floor, open your knees to the corners of your seat, and set your feet back on the floor.

➤ Lift your feet off the floor, bring your knees back in, and return them to the floor.

➤ Repeat for a total of 10.

When you move your knees outward, make sure that your toes point in the same direction as your knees.

10. Seated Leg Lifts with Resistance

➤ Sit in alignment at the front of your chair, feet flat on the floor in front of you.

➤ Place one end of your resistance band on the floor and trap it with your left foot.

➤ Stretch the band around your right thigh and hold it in place with your right hand.

➤ Perform Leg Lifts as usual:

➤ Brace your core.

➤ Lift and lower your right knee 10 times, making sure that the bottom of your foot makes full contact with the floor before you lift again.

➤ Rest.

➤ Repeat with your left knee.

If you don't have a resistance band, perform Seated Leg Lifts as usual, per previous chapters.

Routine 5: Ankle Strengthening Workout

While some of these exercises will be familiar, when you do this workout, focus on your ankle strength and flexibility. I will provide some pointers along the way.

1. Seated March in Place for Ankles

When you do Seated March in Place, you normally lift your foot off the ground and then set the whole thing back down, trying for a good lift of your knees. For the ankle workout, don't worry about lifting your knees high or pumping your arms. When it comes to your feet, you have a choice:

➤ You can lift your feet and just come down lightly on your toes.

➤ You can leave your toes on the floor and just alternate lifting your heels.

Either way, you warm up the flexion in your ankles, which is the goal. March for a count of 20.

2. Seated Heel and Toe Taps

➢ Sit in alignment, feet flat on the floor, hands resting on your thighs.

➢ Lightly brace your core and breathe easily as you extend your right leg with your toes pointing toward the ceiling and tap your heel on the floor.

➢ Bring your right leg back, and lightly tap your toe beneath your chair.

➢ Place your right foot flat on the floor. That was one set.

➢ Repeat with your left foot.

➢ Continue alternating for a count of 10, five sets for each foot.

➢ You are not quite done. You are going to alter the pattern of your taps.

➢ Extend your right leg and set your heel on the floor.

➢ Extend your left leg and set your heel on the floor.

➢ Lift your right foot and bring it back in to rest on the toe near the front of your chair.

➢ Lift your left foot back to meet it. This is one set: right heel/left heel, right toe, left toe.

➢ Continue for a total of 5, counting up each time your right heel goes forward.

3. Gently Point and Flex

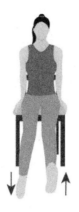 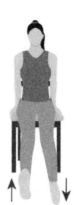

- ➤ Extend both legs so that your heels rest on the floor. Place your hands on the seat behind you if you need extra support.

- ➤ Gently point both toes at the same time.

- ➤ Gently flex both feet at the same time.

- ➤ Continue for a count of 20, counting one for each point and each flex.

- ➤ Change it up and point your right as you flex your left. Think of it as "pump the gas, pump the break."

- ➤ Continue for a count of 20.

Don't strain or try to stretch in your leg muscles. Your goal is to work your ankle flexion.

4. Tap and Rotate

➤ Sit in alignment at the front of your chair, feet flat on the floor, hands on your thighs.

➤ Without raising your foot, gently tap your right toe on the floor 6 times like you are keeping the beat of your favorite song.

➤ Lift your leg and tap 6 more times with your foot in the air.

➤ Keep your leg lifted and rotate your ankle clockwise 4 times.

➤ Rotate it counterclockwise 4 times.

➤ Lower your foot and repeat with your left foot.

5. Extended Rotations

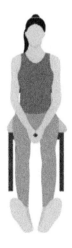 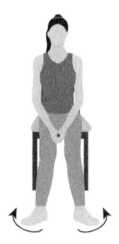

- Sit in alignment, legs extended in front of you, heels resting on the floor, and hands on your thighs.

- Point the toes of both feet.

- Rotate your feet out to the sides away from each other.

- Pull them back into an easy flex while they are still rotated out.

- Bring them back up so that the toes point toward the ceiling.

- Repeat 4 times.

- Reverse the rotation: point, rotate your feet in so that your big toes point toward each other, flex them gently while rotated, return them to starting position.

- Repeat 4 times.

1. **Easy Heel Raises**

- Stand behind your chair in alignment, hands on the chair's back for balance.

- Gently and slowly rise up on your toes and then bring your heels back to the floor.

- Repeat for a total of 10.

- Alter your position by bringing your heels together and turning your toes out to a 45° angle.

- Lift up on your toes for a total of 10.

- Alter your position by bringing your toes together and your heels out.

- Lift up on your toes for another 10.

- Keep the movement slow, smooth, and easy.

This is great for balance, too!

2. **Modified Reverse Lunge**

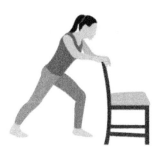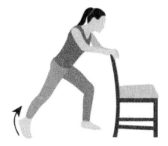

- Stand in alignment behind your chair, hands on the chair's back for support.

- Take a good-sized step back with your right foot (but only about half as far as for Reverse Lunges, Chapter 5), bending your left knee to allow the movement.

- Gently and slowly lift and lower your right heel for a count of 4. It is best to do this by bending and straightening your right knee.

➤ Counter stretch by bending your right knee, straightening your left knee, and flexing your left foot. Push your hips back until you feel a slight stretch in your left calf. Hold for a count of 4.

➤ That was one set: lunge back, pulse your heel 4 times, counter stretch and count 4.

➤ Complete a total of 4 sets on each leg.

As with all of the exercises in this workout, don't try for a major stretch in the calf. Save that for the leg strengthening workout. Your goal here is flexion and blood flow.

Fun fact: the counter stretch is the same position as an Elizabethan courtier's bow!

3. **Advanced Heel Raises**

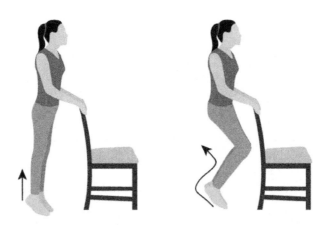

- ➢ Stand in alignment behind your chair, hands on the back for support. Brace your core.

- ➢ Rise up on your toes.

- ➢ While you are on your toes, bend your knees and sink your hips.

- ➢ Still in that position, lower your heels to the floor.

- ➢ Return to standing.

- ➢ Repeat for a total of 5.

- ➢ Reverse the movement:

- ➢ From standing, bend your knees with your feet flat on the floor.

- ➢ Keeping your knees bent, rise up on your toes.

- ➢ Once on your toes, push up and stand straight up on your tippy toes.

- ➢ Return your heels to the floor.

- ➢ Repeat for a total of 5.

Now that your ankle joints are all warmed up, this exercise does actively work the leg muscles. And how!

4. **Calf Stretch**

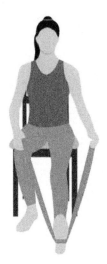 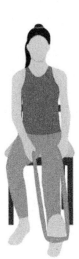

This is good for your ankle and also stretches all of the muscles in your calves. You will need a long, sturdy piece of fabric. Either a necktie or a towel will do the trick.

➢ Sit in alignment at the front of your chair and loop the fabric around the ball of your right foot.

➢ Lift your right foot straight out in front of you, toes pointing toward the ceiling. Choke up on the fabric with both hands, and relax (but don't lock!) your leg.

➢ Using both hands equally, pull straight back on the fabric. You will feel a nice stretch in the large calf muscle group just below your knee.

➢ Hold for 3 full exhales.

➤ Relax for a couple of breaths with your relaxed leg still extended.

➤ Pull with your right hand and encourage your pinky toe to rotate back toward your ear. Feel the stretch in the long, thin muscle that extends from beneath your knee down to your outside ankle.

➤ Hold for 3 exhales.

➤ Relax for a couple of breaths, leg still extended.

➤ Pull with your left hand and encourage your big toe to rotate toward your ear. You will feel the stretch in the inside of your ankle.

➤ Repeat on the left leg.

With your foot in the air, relax your leg. Let your leg be passive and accomplish the stretches using the pressure of the fabric and the strength in your arms.

Remember to position the fabric at the ball of your foot.

Monitor your alignment as you hold and breathe.

➤ Keeping the fabric in place, lower your left foot to the ground and rest on your heel.

➤ Repeat the series of pulls, middle-outside-inside, with your heel on the floor.

➤ Allow your ankle to rotate right and left as you do the inside and outside pulls.

➤ Repeat on the right leg.

If you experience any ankle pain, ease your pull back to that point just before you feel the pain. You can still do the exercise; however, only flex or rotate as far as you can with no pain. Your flexibility will increase over time.

How are your ankles feeling? Stretched and warm and ready for action? Good job, you!

Conclusion

H ere we are at the end, congratulations! I hope you've found the information valuable and the workouts effective. There are eighteen routines in this book. They target all of the muscles in the body. If you find one that you particularly do not like or think especially difficult, that's probably the one you need most. Now, it's up to you to plan and execute a weekly exercise routine. I recommend that you commit to exercising at least three to four days a week. You can mix and match the routines to build your own personal plan. For example:

Week 1

Day 1

➢ Warmup

➢ Seated Core Exercises

➢ Cardio Workout

➢ Hand, Wrist, and Elbow Exercises

Day 2

> Warmup

> Gentle Back Workout

> Belly Fat Exercises

> Legs, Hips, and Balance

Day 3

> Seated Hip Workout

> Standing Arm Toner

> Ankle Strengthening Workout

Notice that after one week, we haven't even used all of the routines yet! There is lots of room for mixing and matching, but follow these guidelines:

1. First, start with a warmup. Some of the routines allow you to skip the warm up in Chapter 2. This is stated at the beginning of those routines.

2. Second, choose a medium intensity routine that targets a specific muscle group.

3. Third, do one of the cardio routines or one of the routines that you know gets your heartrate up.

4. Finish with a low-intensity routine.

This basically amounts to: warm up—work hard—work harder—cool down. Every body is different. As you work through the routines, you will find which are easier for you, which are harder for you, and which really get your heart going. Use this knowledge and experience to customize your own personal plan!

Defeating sarcopenia is all about muscle: feeding muscle, stretching muscle, and building muscle. With the proper diet, lots of water, and regular exercise, I know you are on your way to getting stronger, feeling better, and saying goodbye to chronic pain.

And now, if you'll excuse me, I need to go and do some exercise myself, feeling motivated!

P.S. If you enjoyed the book and found it useful, I would love to read your review on Amazon. Honestly, it's like Christmas morning when I see that someone has enjoyed my book! So thank you in advance.

I intend this to be the first in a series of books for seniors, and I hope you'll keep an eye out for those as I get them finished and available. Thanks so much!

A FREE GIFT TO ALL MY READERS!

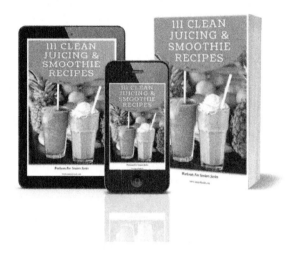

As a thank you, and to help you combine healthy nutrition with your exercise routines to maximize your results, I would like to send you a free copy of my fully illustrated eBook which contains 111 delicious juice and smoothie recipes that you can make at home!

To get your free copy now, please visit:

www.ianneckhardt.com

References

6. Priority diseases and reasons for inclusion 6.24 Low back pain. (n.d.). WHO. https://www.who.int/medicines/areas/priority_medicines/Ch6_24LBP.pdf

24 Hour Home Care. (2015, May 19). Physical therapy exercises for seniors: Shoulder pain relief. Youtube. https://www.youtube.com/watch?app=desktop&v=x1HxcIakOMs

Barnett, B. (n.d.). Is it better to drink cold water while exercising? WebMD. https://www.webmd.com/fitness-exercise/features/is-it-better-to-drink-cold-water-while-exercising

Bed rest for back pain? A little bit will do you. (2015, February 26). Harvard Health. https://www.health.harvard.edu/pain/bed-rest-for-back-pain-a-little-bit-will-do-you

Burgess, L. (2018, April 25). 11 functions of the muscular system: Diagrams, facts, and structure. https://www.medicalnewstoday.com/articles/321617

Cleveland Clinic. (2018, March 28). Joint pain: Symptoms, causes, and treatment. Cleveland Clinic. https://my.clevelandclinic.org/health/symptoms/17752-joint-pain

Cleveland Clinic. (2020, July 13). 5 best ways to safeguard your joints as you age. Health Essentials from Cleveland Clinic. https://health.clevelandclinic.org/5-best-ways-to-safeguard-your-joints-as-you-age

Core stability. (2010). Physiopedia. https://www.physio-pedia.com/Core_stability

Dunkin, Mary Ann. (2009, October). Sarcopenia with aging. WebMD. https://www.webmd.com/healthy-aging/guide/sarcopenia-with-aging

Eldergym Fitness for Seniors. (2020, July 28). Shoulder exercises for seniors. Youtube. https://www.youtube.com/watch?app=desktop&v=CtV7QrKsnlI

Everyday Wellness. (2019, March 15). 4 unexpected benefits of chest exercises.
https://www.everydaywellness.org/community-health/blog/4-unexpected-benefits-of-chest-exercises

Exercise and activity in pain management. (n.d.). Physiopedia. Retrieved July 26, 2021, from
https://www.physio
pedia.com/Exercise_and_Activity_in_Pain_Management#cite_note-p3-7

fabulous50s. (2020, April 17). 10 minute tone your arm workout for women over 50.
Youtube.
https://www.youtube.com/watch?app=desktop&v=8E7cjvOit64

Fitness With Cindy. (2019, September 18). Ankle strengthening exercises for seniors.
Youtube.
https://www.youtube.com/watch?app=desktop&v=xot4AOIeMql

Harvard Health Publishing. (2016, February 19). Preserve your muscle mass.
Harvard Health. https://www.health.harvard.edu/staying-healthy/preserve-your-muscle-mass

Harvard Health Publishing. (2018, November 7). Foods that fight inflammation.
Harvard Health. https://www.health.harvard.edu/staying-healthy/foods-that-fight-inflammation

HUR USA. (n.d.). The truth about exercise after 70. Retrieved July 27, 2021, from
https://blog.hurusa.com/exercise-after-70

Mayo Clinic Staff. (2017a). Core exercises: Why you should strengthen your core muscles.
https://www.mayoclinic.org/healthy-lifestyle/fitness/in-depth/core-exercises/art-20044751

Mayo Clinic Staff. (2017b). Stretching is not a warm up! Find out why.
https://www.mayoclinic.org/healthy-lifestyle/fitness/in-depth/stretching/art-20047931

Mayo Clinic Staff. (2020, February 5). Aerobic exercise: Top 10 reasons to get physical.
https://www.mayoclinic.org/healthy-lifestyle/fitness/in-depth/aerobic-exercise/art-20045541

Milly, H. (2020, May 5). Lift and firm your breasts in 3 weeks.
Youtube.
https://www.youtube.com/watch?app=desktop&v=E1neQOtl4l8

More Life Health Seniors. (2017, July 15). Leg strengthening exercises for seniors:
Decrease knee pain. Youtube. https://www.youtube.com/watch?app=desktop&v=l7L5KUIHnic

More Life Health Seniors. (2018a, August 5). Simple seated core strengthening workout for seniors. Youtube. https://www.youtube.com/watch?v=6Ts-deSDnRM

More Life Health Seniors. (2018b, October 28). Seated hip exercises for seniors.
Youtube. https://www.youtube.com/watch?app=desktop&v=ROwj2dNcL6c

More Life Health Seniors. (2018c, November 18). Hand, wrist & elbow exercises for seniors.
Youtube. https://www.youtube.com/watch?app=desktop&v=MB-2Qa8IYqQ

More Life Health Seniors. (2019, August 6). Leg strengthening exercises for seniors.
Youtube. https://www.youtube.com/watch?v=C6iyYHSsvG0

More Life Health Seniors. (2020a, May 8). Arm exercises for seniors. Youtube. https://www.youtube.com/watch?app=desktop&v=YaM1_I8omDw

More Life Health Seniors. (2020b, May 15). Simple shoulder exercises for seniors.
Youtube. https://www.youtube.com/watch?app=desktop&v=3r-TVaYpAzg

Nagamatsu, L. S. (2012). Resistance training promotes cognitive and functional brain
plasticity in seniors with probable mild cognitive impairment. Archives of Internal Medicine, 172(8), 666. https://doi.org/10.1001/archinternmed.2012.379

Pain Relief Institute. (2019, March 20). Shoulder exercises for seniors. https://www.painfreepainrelief.com/shoulder-exercises-for-seniors/

Sarcopenia. (n.d.). Physiopedia. https://www.physio-pedia.com/Sarcopenia?utm_source=physiopedia&utm_medium=search&utm_campaign=ongoing_internal

Senior Fitness with Meredith. (2019, December 1). Senior fitness low impact cardio workout. Youtube. https://www.youtube.com/watch?app=desktop&v=aViIzXtqi8c

Silver Sneakers. (2020, June 18). 5 exercises for seniors to lose belly fat. Youtube. https://www.youtube.com/watch?app=desktop&v=GQvhi408vAA

Thieme, T. (2021, January 25). Your core muscles are more than just abs. Men's Health. https://www.menshealth.com/fitness/a35307843/core-muscles/

U.S. Department of Health and Human Services. (2019). Physical activity guidelines for Americans 2nd edition. https://health.gov/sites/default/files/2019-09/Physical_Activity_Guidelines_2nd_edition.pdf#page=66

Vive Health. (2020, April 13). 10-minute core workout for seniors. Youtube. https://www.youtube.com/watch?app=desktop&v=H1XLvGWueFs

yes2next. (2020a, July 27). 10-minute leg workout for seniors. Youtube. https://www.youtube.com/watch?app=desktop&v=60fBjmYOGgw

yes2next. (2020b, November 9). Gentle stretching for seniors. Youtube. https://www.youtube.com/watch?v=kfjVFQWWiZw

yes2next. (2021, February 2). Gentle back workout. Youtube. https://www.youtube.com/watch?app=desktop&v=83tNg1ZDYZ4

Printed in Great Britain
by Amazon

73104187R00133